Speech Pathology Manage
Refractory Cough and Rel

Speech Pathology Management of Chronic Refractory Cough and Related Disorders

Anne E. Vertigan

Peter G. Gibson

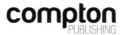
compton
PUBLISHING

Compton Publishing

This edition first published 2016 © 2016 by Compton Publishing Ltd.

Registered office: Compton Publishing Ltd, 30 St. Giles', Oxford, OX1 3LE, UK
Registered company number: 07831037

Editorial offices: 35 East Street, Braunton, EX33 2EA, UK
Web: www.comptonpublishing.co.uk

ISBN 978-1-909082-17-5 (Print edition)

ISBN 978-1-909082-54-0 (Kindle edition)

A catalogue record for this book is available from the British Library.

Cover image: Courtesy Can Stock Photo Inc., www.canstockphoto.com

Cover design: David Siddall, www.davidsiddall.com

Set in Adobe Caslon Pro 12pt by Suart Brown

1   2016

Table of contents

List of contributing authors

Kenneth W. Altman, M.D., Ph.D., FACS, Professor and Vice Chair for Clinical Affairs, The Bobby R. Alford Department of Otolaryngology-Head & Neck Surgery, and Director, The Institute for Voice and Swallowing Baylor College of Medicine, Houston, TX, USA.

Peter G. Gibson, MB BS (Hons), FRACP, F ThorSoc., Senior Staff Specialist, Department of Respiratory and Sleep Medicine, John Hunter Hospital, and Conjoint Professor, Centre for Asthma and Respiratory Diseases, School of Medicine and Public Health, University of Newcastle, Australia.

Marc Haxer, M.A., CCC-SLP, Senior Speech Pathologist, Departments of Speech Pathology and Otolaryngology, University of Michigan Health System, Ann Arbor, MI, USA.

Thomas Murry, Ph.D., FASHA, Professor of Speech Pathology, Department of Otolaryngology-Head and Neck Surgery, Loma Linda Medical University, and co-Director, Loma Linda Voice and Swallowing Center, Loma Linda, CA, USA.

Anne E. Vertigan, B.AppSc(SpPath), MBA, Ph.D., Director, Department of Speech Pathology, John Hunter Hospital, and Conjoint Lecturer, School of Humanities and Social Science (Speech Pathology), University of Newcastle, Centre for Asthma and Respiratory Disease, Hunter Medical Research Institute, School of Medicine & Public Health, University of Newcastle, Australia.

Foreword

"I am so frustrated." This is a phrase that we hear very frequently in our clinics when evaluating patients with chronic cough. It is also frequently mentioned by our colleagues, health care professionals in many specialties who often feel helpless when treating these patients. This welcome book alleviates the frustration as it helps to provide a better understanding of the diagnosis and treatment of this condition, the cough that has no clear etiology, the cough that persists after most common causes of cough have been ruled out, the cough that lingers for years after traditional medical management options have been exhausted.

Imagine yourself avoiding going out to a restaurant or to a movie, missing important family gatherings, staying home instead of going out with friends, being embarrassed to go to church. Imagine further, having coughing fits so strong that your chest hurts from breaking a rib, fear of becoming incontinent, throwing up, or passing out, often without triggers or knowing how to prevent it. This is the reality that countless patients who suffer from chronic refractory cough, their families and coworkers experience on a daily basis. This condition can become debilitating, leading to depression and social isolation. The healthcare community is often at a loss to understand the causes and provide relief to patients who suffer from it.

The last decade has seen a surge in the interest in this type of cough, from research attempting to better characterize the pathophysiology, to development of new therapeutic modalities, including drug trials and behavioral interventions. Anne Vertigan and Peter Gibson have been at the forefront of this important work.

I met Anne Vertigan at the Chronic Cough Conference in New York in 2013, and later at the 2nd Australasian and Asia Pacific Laryngology Congress in Hobart, Australia. I was impressed with her body of work, and appreciated her passion for the pursuit of answers to help cough patients. She has highlighted the critical role of Speech Pathology in the evaluation and treatment of patients with chronic cough and related conditions.

Speech Pathologists are now routinely key players in interdisciplinary teams and work closely with allergy, pulmonary and ear, nose and throat specialists interested in these patients. This collaboration is due in no small part because of Anne Vertigan's work.

The nature of the book is comprehensive. It summarizes the current understanding of the pathophysiology of laryngeal conditions that include refractory cough, laryngeal hypersensitivity and hyperreactivity, and paradoxical vocal fold motion. It includes the perspectives from pulmonary and ear-nose and throat specialties, covers current treatment modalities, and highlights a detailed protocol for behavioral treatment of these disorders. The group of collaborators is top notch, and all share a similar interest and dedication in expanding knowledge and evidence based approaches for cough management.

To date, there have been few resources to help Speech Pathologists who have an interest in chronic cough. This book fills this void. I am sure it will become the reference standard for years to come. It clearly achieves its goal to describe and define chronic refractory cough, to help clinicians in their interdisciplinary efforts to address the condition, and most importantly, to provide Speech Pathologists with a comprehensive guide to understand and treat this difficult patient population.

Claudio F. Milstein Ph.D.
Director, The Voice Center and Section-Head, Division of Speech Language Pathology, Head and Neck Institute, Cleveland Clinic.
Associate Professor of Surgery, Cleveland Clinic Learner School of Medicine.

Preface

We started working with patients with chronic refractory cough and paradoxical vocal fold movement over twenty years ago. At that stage, there was little published information about speech pathology treatment for these conditions, with the majority of the evidence reported in small case series. In fact, we even questioned whether speech pathology treatment was appropriate for these patients.

Over the last twelve years, there has been growing interest amongst speech pathologists in the assessment and treatment of these conditions and an expansion in the evidence for successful treatment. While management of patients with chronic refractory cough is an expanding area of speech-language pathology practice, clinical exposure to the treatment of this condition is variable. Details regarding the theory and treatment of chronic cough have been published in several different fields including respiratory physiology, respiratory medicine, speech pathology, and otolaryngology. This book aims to consolidate this information in order to inform speech pathologists who manage patients with chronic refractory cough and related laryngeal conditions.

This work has developed from our own clinical research and experience working with patients who have chronic refractory cough, however we are constantly learning from other clinicians and researchers as new developments are made in the treatment of these conditions. Three renowned authors, Tom Murry, Ken Altman and Marc Haxer, have contributed chapters to this textbook.

This book has been designed to assist speech pathologists managing patients with chronic refractory cough from the receipt of the initial referral, through to discharge. The book combines theoretical information about cough, with practical advice and tools. The first seven chapters of the book describe the physiology of cough, medical treatment, related laryngeal conditions and hypersensitivity. The remaining chapters describe the treatment approach for speech pathology management of chronic refractory cough and related laryngeal conditions. Although it may be tempting to begin reading this book with assessment and treatment chapters, we believe that it is beneficial to commence with the earlier chapters in order to understand the etiology and physiology of cough and associated medical conditions prior to commencing treatment. It is hoped that this information will make speech pathology treatment for chronic refractory cough more accessible for patients.

This work has only been made possible with the support of our colleagues. We would particularly like to acknowledge the invaluable assistance of Sarah Kapela, speech pathologist at John Hunter Hospital, for her invaluable work as a research assistant and for advice regarding photography and layout. There are several other people we would like to thank, including Dr Josephine Smith from the University of Newcastle for her expertise in cranial nerves, Sienna Tuckerman, speech pathologist at John Hunter Hospital for assistance regarding cough physiology, Mark Rothfield from the Hunter Medical Research Institute, and Mary Aldrich and for photography and formatting. We would like to thank the Hunter New England Speech Pathology Evidence Based Practice group for designing the format upon which we based our clinical observation form. We appreciate the assistance of Professor Deborah Theodoros and Dr Alison Winkworth for their expertise in supervising the early research that under-pinned this work. We would like to thank our colleagues in speech pathology, respiratory medicine and otolaryngology at John Hunter Hospital who have provided ongoing support and continued to raise questions to expand the work in this important area. Finally we would like to thank our patients who have taught us so much over the years.

Dr. Anne Vertigan
Prof. Peter Gibson

Dedicated to Jennifer Thomas, whose generosity in providing a grant to support our initial research has led to the development of our treatment program and paved the way for new developments in the field.

1

Introduction

Coughing is such a common experience that it in fact accounts for the largest number of outpatient health care visits.[1,2] Yet because most cases of acute cough resolve spontaneously or with a single course of medical treatment, we barely give it a second thought. But chronic cough is another matter. This is defined as a cough that lasts for longer than eight weeks, and it is a significant health problem for many people.[1] Often lasting for months or even years, chronic cough has debilitating side effects including stress urinary incontinence, depression, poor sleep, headaches and reduced quality of life.[3,4] Some patients resign from work. Many avoid social situations. Even simple activities such as conversing or using the telephone can become distressing because talking can trigger coughing episodes.[5]

The history of cough

The recent history of cough in the modern medical era was succinctly described by Song.[6] Cough was previously thought to be associated with respiratory infection and chronic bronchitis resulting from transmitted infection, or exposure to airborne pollutants or tobacco smoke. It was subsequently found that not all patients fitted the respiratory infection paradigm and that cough may be due to other diseases such as asthma, rhinitis, and gastroesophageal reflux disease.

In 1990, Irwin[7,8] described the Anatomic Diagnostic Protocol. This protocol recognised the wide sensory distribution of the vagus nerve, and proposed that sensory stimulation of any of the organs innervated by this nerve could lead to hyperstimulation and cough. This insight was then applied to diagnostics and the goal was to identify the associated disease causing cough in an individual patient. For example, asthma results in airway irritation and cough, rhinitis leads to stimulation of vagal nerve endings in the upper airway, and gastroesophageal reflux causes acid induced esophageal inflammation and neural activation. The result of these diverse diseases is a common pathway of vagal sensory activation and cough. The Anatomic Diagnostic Protocol then directs treatment to the associated disease, as a means to resolve the cough.

This approach was reported to be successful in virtually all cases. Idiopathic or unexplained cough was diagnosed when cough persists despite complete workup and appropriate therapeutic trials.[9] This entity has been questioned as a failure to systematically apply the Anatomic Diagnostic Protocol. However, McGarvey[10] and Haque *et al.*[11] postulated that idiopathic cough was a distinct entity with unknown underlying pathophysiology and no treatment options. Idiopathic cough is more likely preceded by an upper respiratory tract infection, is usually longer duration of cough and shows increased sensitivity to capsaicin.

More recently, in 2010, the notion of Cough Hypersensitivity Syndrome was introduced.[12] This hypothesis views chronic cough as a single syndrome with the underlying etiology of cough hypersensitivity. The Cough Hypersensitivity Syndrome theory reconceptualises commonly associated diseases, such as asthma, which were previously thought to cause cough, as cough triggers in an individual with underlying hypersensitivity. Another concept is the existence of a second lesion which causes cough persistence despite treatment. This could be (1) central sensitisation of the cough reflex, or (2) extrathoracic airway hyper-responsiveness, or both. These paradigm shifts are summarised in Table 1.1.

The role of speech pathology

Speech pathologists have an important role to play in the treatment of patients with chronic cough. It is an emerging area of speech pathology practice that provides a valuable treatment option for patients who may have exhausted medical treatment for their condition. There may also be a role for speech pathologists in non-pharmacological management of cough in a range of other conditions. However, further research is required to establish this.

Speech pathology treatment for chronic cough improves the individual's control over cough, reduces cough symptoms and associated symptoms of dysphonia, and paradoxical vocal fold movement (described in Chapters 7 and 11). This treatment results in improved cough symptom ratings,[13] acoustic and auditory perceptual voice results,[14] cough frequency, and capsaicin cough reflex sensitivity.[15]

	< 1990	1990	2010
Prevailing concept	Cough as a response to environmental irritants.	Stimulation of afferent limb of cough reflex.	1. Central reflex sensitization. 2. Laryngeal hypersensitivity.
Cause	Disease. Infection. Tobacco. Smoke.	Asthma. Gastroesophageal reflux. Rhinosinusitis	Sensory neuropathy Central sensitization
Treatment	Antibiotics. Smoking cessation.	Proton pump inhibitors. Inhaled corticosteroids. Antihistamines. Topical steroids.	Centrally acting neuromodulators. Speech pathology.

Table 1.1: Incremental concept developments in chronic refractory cough

There are several reasons why speech pathology treatment is appropriate for chronic cough. Speech pathology management of chronic cough employs techniques adapted from those used to treat hyperfunctional voice disorders[16,17] and involves teaching individuals over a number of sessions to control a function previously considered automatic and outside of their control. Speech pathology management of hyperfunctional voice disorders is effective in teaching patients to reduce phonotraumatic behaviours such as coughing and throat clearing.[18] This is important because such behaviours may lead to ongoing tissue damage and cough persistence. Other techniques used in the management of chronic cough and paradoxical vocal fold movement have included pitch change, diaphragmatic or abdominal breathing, focusing on expiration, reducing extrinsic muscle tension, relaxation and sniffing to reduce improper vocal fold adduction.[17] Stemple claimed that the combination of a detailed knowledge of the upper airways and proven ability to effect behavioural change make speech pathologists excellent professionals to treat this condition. Speech pathologists have extensive experience in education and training in respiratory physiology and modifying laryngeal behaviour.[19] Mathers-Schmidt[20] argued that the speech pathologist's knowledge in the areas of voice, swallowing, and motor speech disorders prepares clinicians to detect abnormalities in laryngeal and respiratory functions and to teach laryngeal and respiratory control techniques. Finally, laryngeal dysfunction is implicated in the pathogenesis of chronic cough. This concept will be elaborated on in Chapter 7.

The aim and outline of the book

The aim of this book is to equip speech pathologists to manage patients presenting with chronic cough. Management of chronic cough is an expanding area for speech pathologists, yet many have limited clinical exposure to the treatment of this condition. Furthermore, while the comprehensive details of the theory and treatment of chronic cough are known, they have been published in a diverse range of separate documents in the fields of respiratory physiology, respiratory medicine, speech pathology, and otolaryngology, and as such they are not readily available in a combined form. Knowledge of the etiology and physiology of cough and associated medical conditions is essential for speech pathologists.

This book aims to describe the theoretical basis of this growing area of clinical practice, to describe a new approach to the problem, and provide clinicians with tools that can aid their practice. It will outline the assessment and treatment process to manage the condition. While knowledge of voice disorders is invaluable in the treatment of chronic cough, a specific framework for assessing and treating chronic cough is frequently required. These concepts will be outlined in this book.

Laryngeal hypersensitivity is emerging as an important concept in chronic refractory cough. It is the target of mechanisms studies, novel therapies and also novel pharmacological developments. Recently published evidence for laryngeal hypersensitivity in chronic refractory cough will be outlined along with new approaches for measuring this component of the disorder.

Speech pathologists, referring medical specialists and patients have expressed a need for more specialized speech pathology services for the management of chronic cough. In particular, speech pathologists are requesting more comprehensive and cohesive information to guide their patient management. As more speech pathologists are required to treat patients with chronic refractory cough, there is a need for more information regarding treatment of this disorder.

This book describes the pathophysiology of chronic cough and the speech pathology assessment and treatment the condition. The first seven chapters provide theoretical information about chronic cough which is not easily accessible to most speech pathologists. This information includes the definition and clinical presentation of the patient with chronic cough, associated medical conditions and laryngeal disorders associated with chronic refractory cough, and the otolaryngology and respiratory medicine management of the condition. A chapter on pulmonary function testing has been included to assist the speech pathologist interpret and understand pulmonary function test results.

The remaining chapters (8 to 13) include a detailed outline of the speech pathology assessment and treatment of chronic cough. It describes the evidence base for behavioural treatment, detailed instructions regarding selection and use of treatment techniques along with user friendly resources. Information about the management of related laryngeal conditions such as paradoxical vocal fold movement and globus pharyngeus has been included as these conditions frequently co-occur with chronic cough and there are several overlaps in the treatment of the conditions. It may be tempting for the speech pathologist to commence reading at this latter section. However we argue that the speech pathologist should be familiar with the physiology of cough and associated medical conditions in order to effectively treat the conditions. The anatomy and physiology of speech, phonation and respiration at an undergraduate speech pathology level is presumed as is competency in the assessment and treatment of speech, voice and swallowing disorders.

Terminology and definitions

Cough

A cough can be defined as "an airway defensive reflex consisting of an inspiratory phase followed by a forced expiratory effort initially against a closed glottis, followed by active glottal opening and rapid expiratory flow"[21 (page S3)]. Cough has an important role in protecting the airway from foreign bodies and aspiration, removing noxious substances and increasing mucociliary clearance. Cough is particularly important in protecting the airway during swallowing in individuals with aspiration resulting from oropharyngeal dysphagia.

Cough can become a troublesome symptom leading people to seek medical assistance. Under this situation, temporal definitions are applied to the classification of cough, such that cough is defined as acute, or chronic. Cough may also be classified as subacute when it lasts for an intermediate period of time. This classification is more frequently used in paediatrics. It is discussed in more detail in Chapter 5. These terms are generally restricted to clinical definitions such as when cough becomes a symptom that the individual complains about.

Acute cough

An acute cough is defined as a cough that resolves within three weeks.[22] Most cases of acute cough are due to upper or lower respiratory tract infection. These cases may resolve spontaneously or following appropriate pharmacotherapy. Speech pathologists are seldom required to provide intervention for patients with acute cough.

Chronic cough

Chronic cough is simply defined as a cough persisting for longer than eight weeks.[23,9] Chronic dry cough without associated disease is considered to have no benefit to the respiratory system or the body in general.[8] The majority of cases (80%) of chronic cough resolve after medical treatment. Medical treatment for chronic cough typically involves withdrawing Angiotensin Converting Enzyme-I inhibitors, if used, and treating coexisting asthma, gastroesophageal reflux, rhinosinusitus, or lung pathology.

Chronic refractory cough

Chronic refractory cough is a cough that has lasted for longer than eight weeks **and** is refractory to appropriate medical management. While the majority of cases of chronic cough respond to medical management, cough remains refractory to medical treatment in between 12% and 42% of cases.[24,25,11] Some patients with chronic cough fail to respond to medical treatment despite extensive investigation.[26] It is this subset of patients with chronic refractory cough that requires speech pathology intervention.

It is important to distinguish between chronic cough that is responsive to medical treatment and chronic cough that persists despite medical treatment. Figure 1.1 outlines the model for conceptualising cough that does not respond to medical treatment. In this model, cough is classified as either acute or chronic depending upon the duration of symptoms. Chronic cough is then further classified as either cough that responds to medical treatment or cough that is refractory to medical treatment. Cough that fails to respond to medical treatment may be referred to as chronic refractory cough.

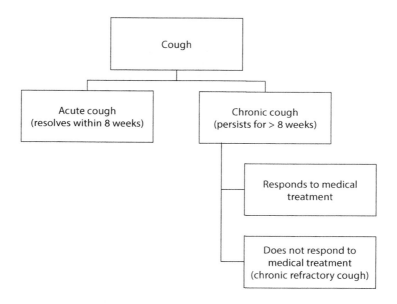

Figure 1.1: Model for the conceptualisation of chronic cough that does not respond to medical intervention.

A variety of terms have been used to describe chronic refractory cough in the literature. These terms include chronic idiopathic cough, chronic unexplained cough, cough hypersensitivity syndrome and chronic non-specific cough. These latter terms suggest that a cause for a cough cannot be found whereas the term chronic refractory cough suggests that the cause for cough is known but it remains refractory to medical treatment.

The difference in terminology makes research and common understanding of the condition difficult. Despite a lack of consensus around terminology be used we have used the term *chronic refractory cough* to refer to cough that has lasted for longer than 8 weeks and which has either no known etiology, or has persisted despite medical management of a known etiology.

Chronic refractory cough may co-occur with paradoxical vocal fold movement and globus pharyngeus.[27] These conditions may be associated with laryngeal dysfunction and have an increased prevalence of impaired laryngeal sensation[28], voice disorders,[29] and paradoxical vocal fold movement. The etiology of chronic refractory cough is unknown. Research has shown it is not responsive to medical treatment including treatment of lung pathology, asthma, rhinosinusitis, and gastroesophageal reflux disease.[11]

7

The burden of cough

Cough accounts for between 10% and 38% of respiratory outpatient visits in the USA.[30] The prevalence of chronic cough varies between studies: in the general population it is between 3% and 33%[30,31,32] and as high as 40% in patients attending specialist cough clinics. In the general population, cough severe enough to interfere with every day activities is estimated to be 7%.[33] Although under-recognised, chronic cough is a significant health problem for many individuals. The incidence of chronic cough and the duration of the condition result in a significant disease burden.

Physical side effects of chronic cough

Physical side effects of cough include syncope, musculoskeletal chest wall pain, headache, difficulty speaking on the telephone, increased pressure on lumbar discs, laryngeal trauma, stress urinary incontinence, fatigue, damage to airway mucosa, exhaustion, vomiting, and rib fractures.[34,35] Although not explicitly studied, cough may also contribute to the development of paradoxical vocal fold movement and laryngeal hypersensitivity.

Quality of life in patients with chronic cough

In addition to physical side effects, cough has a negative impact on quality of life. These effects include disruption to normal activity, interference with work and social relationships, worry about serious medical illness, frequent retching, exhaustion, embarrassment, self-consciousness, social isolation, prolonged frustration, guilt, depression, sleep deprivation, and lethargy.[4,31,36–44] Effective treatment of chronic cough therefore has the potential to significantly improve the quality of everyday life for these patients.

Financial impacts of chronic cough

Chronic refractory cough also has significant financial implications. For the individual patient, the cost of medical consultations along with over the counter and prescribed medications is considerable. Reduced capacity for employment and work attendance can also have financial ramifications for some individuals. At the health service level, the costs of cough are frequently underestimated as patients rarely die and are seldom admitted to hospital. Nevertheless, the cost of physician consultations and emergency department visits is significant. Therefore, it is important to have adequate treatment options available for individuals with chronic refractory cough.

Fortunately, the side effects of chronic cough are often relieved following successful medical treatment of this condition.[4] However when cough persists despite medical treatment, the side effects are likely to continue thus exacerbating the impact of the condition. Further, the pathway to a final diagnosis of chronic refractory cough may be extended, and potentially lead to expensive or inappropriate medical treatments.[45] Murry reports that patients with chronic refractory cough have often been examined by several specialists before commencing speech pathology treatment.

Summary

Chronic cough is a significant clinical problem that is being increasing managed by speech pathologists. Although cough resolves spontaneously or with medical treatment, it persists in a subset of patients. The development of the Anatomic Diagnostic Protocol and Cough Hypersensitivity Syndrome were significant developments in cough, and provided new avenues for the assessment and treatment of patients with the condition. Recently, the role of laryngeal hypersensitivity in cough has been recognised as an important component. These developments are significant as chronic refractory cough is a debilitating condition with significant impacts on quality of life.

References

1. Britt H, Miller G, Knox S, *et al. General Practice Activity in Australia 2003–2004.* Canberra: Australian Institute of Health and Welfare; 2004.

2. Schappert S, Rechtsteiner E. Ambulatory medical care utilization estimates for 2007. National Center for Health Statistics. *Vital Health Stat.* 2011;13(169).

3. Dicipinigaitis P, Tso R, Banauch G. Prevalence of depressive symptoms among patients with chronic cough. *Chest.* 2006;130(6):1839–43.

4. French C, Irwin R, Curley F, Krikorian C. Impact of chronic cough quality of life. *Archives of Internal Medicine.* 1998;158(15):1657–61.

5. Vertigan AE, Gibson PG. Chronic refractory cough as a sensory neuropathy: evidence from a reinterpretation of cough triggers. *Journal of Voice.* 2011;25(5):596–601.

6. Song W-J, Chang Y-S, Morice A. Changing the paradigm for cough: does 'cough hypersensitivity' aid our understanding? *Asia Pacific Allergy.* 2013;4(1):3–13.

7. Irwin R, Curley F, French C. Chronic cough: the spectrum and frequency of causes, key components of the diagnostic evaluation and outcome of specific thearpy. *American Review of Respiratory Disease.* 1990;141:640–7.

8. Irwin R, Boulet L, Cloutier M, *et al.* Managing cough as a defence mechanism and as a symptom: a consensus report for the American College of Chest Physicians. *Chest.* 1998;114(2):133S (47).

9. Pratter M, Brightling C, Boulet L, Irwin R. An empiric integrative approach to the management of cough: ACCP evidence-based clinical practice guidelines. *Chest.* 2006;129(1 Suppl):222S–31S.

10. McGarvey L, Forsythe P, Heaney L, *et al.* Idiopathic chronic cough: a real disease or a failure of diagnosis? *Cough.* 2005;1(9).

11. Haque R, Usmani O, Barnes P. Chronic idiopathic cough: a discrete clinical entity? *Chest.* 2005;127(5):1710–3.

12. Morice A. The cough hypersensitivity syndrome: a novel paradigm for understanding cough. *Lung.* 2010;188(Suppl 1):S87–S90.

13. Vertigan A, Theodoros D, Gibson P, Winkworth A. Efficacy of speech pathology management for chronic cough: a randomised, single blind, placebo controlled trial of treatment efficacy. *Thorax.* 2006;61:1065–9.

14. Vertigan A, Theodoros D, Winkworth A, Gibson P. A comparison of two approaches to the treatment of chronic cough: perceptual acoustic and electroglottographic outcomes. *Journal of Voice.* 2008;22(5):581–9.

15. Ryan NM, Vertigan AE, Bone S, Gibson PG. Cough reflex sensitivity improves with speech language pathology management of refractory chronic cough. *Cough.* 2010;6(1):1–8.

16. Blager F, Gay M, Wood R. Voice therapy techniques adapted to treatment of habit cough: pilot study. *Journal of Communication Disorders.* 1998;21:393–400.

17. Altman K, Mirza N, Ruiz C, Sataloff R. Paradoxical vocal fold motion: presentation and treatment options. *Journal of Voice.* 2000;14(1):99–103.

18. Broaddus-Lawrence P, Treole K, McCabe R, *et al.* The effects of preventive vocal hygiene education on the habits and perceptual vocal characteristics of training singers. *Journal of Voice.* 2000;14(1):68–71.

19. Stemple J, Fry L. *Voice Therapy: Clinical Case Studies.* 3rd edn. San Diego, CA: Plural Publishing; 2009.

20. Mathers-Schmidt B. Paradoxical vocal fold motion: a tutorial on a complex disorder and the speech-language pathologist's role. *American Journal of Speech Language Pathology.* 2001;10:111–25.

21. Fontana GA. Before we get started: what is a cough? *Lung.* 2008;186(1):2.

22. Irwin RS. Introduction to the diagnosis and management of cough : ACCP evidence-based clinical practice guidelines. *Chest.* 2006;129(1 suppl):25S ACCP 7S.

23. McGarvey L. Clinical assessment of cough. In: Chung K, Widdicome J, Boushey H (ed). *Cough: Causes, Mechanisms and Therapy.* Melbourne: Blackwell Publishing; 2003.

24. Ringsberg K, Segesten K, Akerlind I. Walking around in circles – the life situation of patients with asthma-like symptoms but negative asthma tests. *Scandinavian Journal of Caring Sciences.* 1997;11:103–12.

25. Kardos . Proposals for a rationale and for rational diagnosis of cough. *Pneumologie.* 2000;54(3):110–5.

26. Birring S. Controversies in the evaluation and management of chronic cough. *American Journal of Respiratory & Critical Care Medicine.* 2011;183(6):708–15.

27. Ryan N, Gibson P. Characterization of laryngeal dysfunction in chronic persistent cough. *The Laryngoscope.* 2009;119(4):640–5.

28. Vertigan A, Bone S, Gibson PG. Laryngeal sensory dysfunction in laryngeal hypersensitivity syndrome. *Respirology.* 2010;18(6):948–56.

29. Vertigan A, Theodoros D, Winkworth A, Gibson P. Perceptual voice characteristics in chronic cough and paradoxical vocal fold movement. *Folia Phoniatrica et Logopaedica.* 2007;59(5):256–67.

30. Chung KF, Pavord ID. Prevalence, pathogenesis, and causes of chronic cough. *The Lancet.* 2008;371(9621):1364–74.

31. Chamberlain SA, Garrod R, Douiri A, *et al.* The impact of chronic cough: a cross-sectional European survey. *Lung.* 2015;193(3):401–8.

32. Marchant JM, Newcombe PA, Juniper EF, *et al.* What is the burden of chronic cough for families? *Chest.* 2008;134(2):303–9.

33. Ford AC, Forman D, Moayyedi P, Morice AH. Cough in the community: a cross sectional survey and the relationship to gastrointestinal symptoms. *Thorax* 2006;61(11):975–9.

34. McGarvey L, McKeagney P, Polley L, *et al.* Are there clinical features of a sensitized cough reflex? *Pulmonary Pharmacology & Therapeutics.* 2009;22:59–64.

35. Morice A, McGarvey L, Dicipinigaitis P. Cough hypersensitivity syndrome is an important clinical concept: a pro/con debate. *Lung.* 2011;190(1):3–9.

36. Shuttari M, Braun S. Contemporary management of chronic persistent cough. *Missouri Medicine.* 1992;89(11):795–800.

37. Reigel B, Warmoth J, Middaugh S, *et al.* Psychogenic cough treated with biofeedback and psychotherapy: a review and case report. *American Journal of Physical Medical Rehabilitation.* 1995;74(2):155–8.

38. Kelsey J. An epidemiological study of acute herniated lumbar intervertebral discs. *Rheumatology & Rehabilitation.* 1975;14(3):144–59.

39. Ward P, Zwitman D, Hanson D, Berci G. Contact ulcers and granulomas of the larynx: new insights into their etiology as a basis for more rational treatment. *Otolaryngology Head & Neck Surgery.* 1980;88(3):262–9.

11

40. DelDonno M, Aversa C, Corsico R, *et al*. Efficacy and safety of moguisterine in comparison with dextromethorphan in patients with persistent cough. *Drug Investigation*. 1994;7(2):92–100.

41. Miller J. On pelvic floor muscle function and stress urinary incontinence: effects of posture, parity and volitional control. Ph.D. Dissertation. Michigan: University of Michigan; 1996.

42. Mazzone S, Canning B, Widdicome J. Sensory pathways for the cough reflex. In: Chung K, Widdicome J, Boushey H (eds). *Cough: Causes, Mechanisms and Therapy*. Melbourne: Blackwell Publishing; 2003.

43. Bunyavejchevin S. Risk factors of female urinary incontinence and overactive bladder in Thai postmenopausal women. *Journal of the Medical Association of Thailand*. 2005;88(4):S119–23.

44. Hanak V, Hartman T, Rye J. Cough-induced rib fractures. *Mayo Clinic Proceedings*. 2005;80(7):879–82.

45. Milgrom H, Corsello P, Freedman M, *et al*. Differential diagnosis and management of chronic cough. *Comprehensive Therapy*. 1990;16(10):46–53.

2

Physiology of cough

Anne E. Vertigan and Peter G. Gibson

The assessment and treatment of chronic refractory cough should be designed with an appreciation of the physiology of cough. Significant developments in the understanding of cough physiology are derived from the field of respiratory physiology. There is a remarkable consistency between this work and developments in the field of speech pathology. This chapter describes several issues relating to cough physiology including the type of cough, urge to cough and neurophysiology of cough. Several types of cough and throat clearing have been described in the literature and understanding these has relevance for the behavioural management of chronic refractory cough. The Urge to Cough model provides an understanding of the process from exposure to a cough trigger to the execution of the cough. Finally the neurophysiology of cough is also relevant to understanding sensory activation of the cough reflex, and the role of central neural sensitisation, particularly as it applies to chronic refractory cough.

Cough is a protective mechanism and represents the outcome of a complex reflex, initiated by activation of irritant receptors in the airway.[1,2] There are three phases to cough: inspiration, compression and expulsion. Cough is essential for airway protection but can become harmful when it becomes excessive. The cough is produced with high intrathoracic pressure (300mmHg) and velocity up to 800 km/hour.[3]

Type of cough

Cough may be either voluntary or reflexive. Although not strictly a cough, throat clearing and the expiratory reflex may serve a similar benefit to the airway and have been included in this discussion.

Voluntary cough

Voluntary cough originates in the cerebral cortex and involves an intention to cough.[4] It may occur when an individual decides to cough to clear irritation from their throat or when they are asked to cough. Voluntary cough is not produced by the motor centre. It is assessed clinically by asking the patient to cough. An individual who is conscious, but cannot respond to a request for voluntary cough may have damage to the cortical descending pathways for cough but have an intact reflexive cough.

Reflexive cough

Reflexive cough follows a similar pattern to voluntary cough but has different neurological pathways. In reflexive cough, several glottal closures and expiratory efforts may be contained in one cough. Objective assessment of reflexive cough requires administering a known tussive stimulant, such as capsaicin, and measuring the response, for example the number of coughs produced. Reflexive cough is caused by direct activation of receptors on airway sensory nerves.[5] The neurophysiology of reflexive cough differs from that of voluntary cough.

Expiratory reflex

In addition to voluntary and reflexive cough, respiratory physiologists also describe the expiratory reflex.[6] The expiratory reflex is stimulated when solid, liquid or chemical irritation touches the true vocal folds or upper tracheal areas and results in prompt closure of glottis by contraction of the laryngeal adductor muscles, with strong expiratory effort by contraction of the expiratory muscles, followed by opening of glottis and expulsion of air from lungs.[7] The expiratory reflex starts with vocal fold closure and expiration, and the function is to prevent aspiration. Although the expiratory reflex does not commence with inspiration, inspiration can commence later. In contrast, both voluntary and reflexive cough start with inspiration, and the function is to draw air into the lungs to promote a more efficient subsequent expulsion of mucous and airway debris. The expiratory reflex can be voluntary such as that which occurs during throat clearing.

There is a clear and significant physiological difference between cough and the expiratory reflex. Despite this difference, there is often limited differentiation between these two reflexes in the speech pathology management of oropharyngeal dysphagia. In clinical practice it is presumed that a cough is physiologically required to protect the airway. Yet the respiratory physiology literature argues that it is the expiratory reflex rather than a cough reflex that protects the airway. In other words, 'cough' occurring during tracheal aspiration is probably the laryngeal expiratory reflex rather than reflexive cough, as reflexive cough would commence with inspiration and draw food and fluids further into the lungs.[4]

Throat clearing

Throat clearing is distinct from cough and can be reflexive or voluntary. Throat clearing does not have an inspiratory phase. Throat clearing may serve several functions. It may occur in response to irritation in the laryngeal region. Even though throat clearing is a phonotraumatic behaviour, some individuals use it to initiate phonation particularly when there is difficulty with voice onset. Deliberate throat clearing can also be used to add effect during communication, for example to gain somebody's attention.

Urge to Cough model

The concept of the Urge to Cough is important in the assessment and management of chronic refractory cough. The Urge to Cough model can be used as a basis for the assessment and treatment of the patient with chronic refractory cough.[8] The urge to cough precedes the cough motor response.[9] There is a relationship between the magnitude estimation of the urge to cough and cough reflex sensitivity as measured by capsaicin.[10] The magnitude of the Urge to Cough can be reliably estimated by the patient using the scale shown in Table 2.1, however some patients may find it difficult to separate the Urge to Cough from the cough motor response.[9] In these urge to cough ratings, the patient indicates the number that correlates to their perceived Urge to Cough. The magnitude of the Urge to Cough is not static and can be influenced by several internal and external factors.

In addition to estimating the magnitude of the Urge to Cough, Davenport developed a six stage model to describe the urge to cough.[10] The six stages are (1) stimulus, (2) urge, (3) desire, (4) action, i.e. cough, (5) feedback, and (6) reward.

These stages are outlined in the following sections. The Urge to Cough model is significant in understanding the physiology of cough. The principles in the Urge to Cough model are relevant to the management of conditions such as chronic refractory cough and paradoxical vocal fold movement.

Rating	Description
0	Nothing at all
0.5	Very, very weak (just noticeable)
1	Very weak
2	Weak
3	Moderate
4	Somewhat strong
5	Strong
6	
7	Very strong
8	
9	
10	Very very strong (almost maximum)

Table 2.1: Urge to Cough scale.[11]

Stage one: cough stimulus

The cough stimulus is the trigger for a neural event. The mechanical or sensory stimuli triggers cough receptors in the airway and projects to neural structures. In a patient with chronic cough, the stimulus causes activation of the airway nerves but with no airway compromise or functional need to clear the airway.

Stage two: urge

The urge is the physical need to respond to the stimulus. In this stage, the physical stimulus is converted into a biological urge. The thalamus transfers the sensory urge to the limbic system. In a patient with chronic refractory cough, this stimulus creates an urge to cough even when there is nothing to clear from the airway. In other words, the urge to cough is hypersensitive.

Stage three: desire

The desire is the translation of the urge into a central neural targeted goal. This process involves cortical activation. It produces a conscious motivation to cough or to suppress a cough. If sufficient, the urge may overcome the desire to suppress the cough. During the desire stage, the individual will perceive a need to clear irritation from their airway.

Stage four: action

The action is the physical response that satisfies the urge-desire. The action results from descending cortical motor drive that activates the brain stem cough control network which subsequently generates the cough. The individual makes a physical response to either cough or to suppress their cough. Either way they will satisfy the urge-desire. Most patients with chronic refractory cough will have a dry and non-productive cough. In some cases the patient may even cough deliberately to clear the irritation from their throat or may cough repeatedly in attempt to clear minute quantities of secretion. This cough behaviour can increase sensitivity and irritation in the airway and lead to phonotrauma.

Stage five: feedback

The feedback system stimulated by the cough provides the central nervous system with evidence that the cough has occurred or been suppressed. Feedback comes from cough sensory receptors and central neurological centres. The individual receives feedback that the cough has been relieved and that the irritation has been temporarily relieved. This behaviour may, however, form a cycle where irritation leads to coughing, which creates further irritation that subsequently leads to further coughing.

Stage six: reward

The reward is the sensory system that determines whether or not the urge was satisfied. In other words, it is the affective reward for action. Feedback is projected via a limbic system which mediates the sense of reward. The brain provides cognitive information that the appropriate action has occurred – either that the cough needs to continue or that it could cease.

Neurophysiology of cough

The neurophysiology of cough is extremely complex. An in-depth understanding of the neurophysiology may help the speech pathologist appreciate why the individual patient is coughing and the mechanism underlying the cough behaviour. Many speech pathologists attribute neurological control of cough as being mediated by the vagus nerve and are particularly interested in in its function during dysphagia management. In the management of chronic refractory cough, additional concepts including cough stimuli, airway afferent nerves, and central processing are relevant.

Coughing is usually the result of an involuntary reflex response to stimulation of vagal afferent nerves in pulmonary and extrapulmonary sites in the airways.[3,12,13] Activation of these vagal afferent sensory nerves projects a signal centrally to the nucleus tractus solitarius in the medulla.[13] The signal then undergoes modulation which generates a motor response.[13] While cough is a visceral reflex, it also has higher cortical control[13] and, similar to other reflexes such as swallowing and urinating, it can be voluntarily inhibited or initiated.[3, 13–16] The complexities of these processes are explored in the following sections of this chapter.

Cough stimuli

Airway afferent nerves can be irritated by both chemical and mechanical stimuli[3] and result in cough. The basic primary defensive cough reflex is caused by mechanical stimulation such as aspiration, foreign body inhalation or direct mechanical probing of the airway mucosa. In contrast, cough associated with chronic airway irritation, airway obstruction and substances such as capsaicin, adenosine, bradykinin and citric acid, is stimulated by chemosensor pathways.[17] These chemical stimuli evoke cough in conscious individuals but not in unconscious individuals even though the cough can be stimulated by touching airway mucosa.[17] Therefore cough stimulated by chemical stimuli may not necessarily be reflexive as it requires the individual to be conscious, and suggests that the perception of airway irritation and an urge to cough is an essential component of cough triggered by chemical stimuli.

Transient Receptor Potentials

Transient Receptor Potentials (TRP) are ion channels found on the cell membrane in mammals. Knowledge of TRP receptors is not essential for the behavioural management of cough but may be of interest to speech pathologists who wish to explore cough physiology in more detail. TRP receptors mediate sensations such as pain and temperature and play a vital role in the modulation of cough. The two most important TRP receptors in the modulation of cough are the Transient Receptor Potential Vanilloid (TRPV1) and the Transient Receptor Potential Ankrin (TRPA1). These TRP receptors are expressed on the C-Fibres of airway afferent nerves[18] and evoke painful and noxious sensations and reflexes.[13] These receptors are increased in patients with chronic refractory cough. Upregulation of TRP nociceptors leads to upper airway hypersensitivity.

TRPV1 are present on airway sensory nerves in the trachea, bronchi and nasal mucosa. They are activated by capsaicin (the pungent part of chilli) and painfully hot stimuli > 40°C. TRPV1 mediate inflammation and thermal hyperalgesia.[18]

TRPA1 are activated by allyl isothiocynate (mustard oil) which is the pungent part of wasabi or mustard. It is also activated by cinnamaldehyde allicin (cinnamon), and diallyl sulphides (from garlic and onion). More recent studies have identified a broad range of chemicals that activate TRPA1. TRPA1 may have an important role in the development of prolonged cough. TRPA1 agonist activation depends on the reversible or irreversible nature of the chemical bonds formed on membrane permeability.[18] Glutathione levels can affect the potency of inhaled airway irritants and once these levels are depleted, TRPA1 may act more intensely. Prolonged exposure to the stimulus may heighten TRPA1 activity in a cumulative fashion. Channels may become irreversibly modified and stay active for long periods of time. Cross stimulation of TRPA1 activity may continue and explain why a prolonged sensation of irritation is present even when the noxious stimuli is removed.[18]

TRPA1 function is dependent upon calcium ions (Ca^{2+}). Studies have found that when Ca^{2+} is removed then TRPA1 reacts less strongly than if Ca^{2+} is present. Therefore Ca^{2+} has a major role in stimulation. There is an influx of Ca^{2+} through the channel pore which increases intracellular Ca^{2+}. This mechanism can disconnect the TRPA1 activity from the initial stimulus.[18] The result of the disconnection is that TRPA1 channels in the region of the activated channels may become activated.[18] For example, reflux may stimulate certain TRPA1 channels after which TRPA1 channels in another region also become activated simply by a spill over of Ca^{2+}, even though not in direct contact with the stimulus. TRPA1 may also amplify other Ca^{2+} pathways, including TRPV1, or release Ca^{2+} from intracellular stores. This process of amplification leads to neuronal excitation and local inflammatory release of neuropeptides. Recruitment of additional fibres, can lead to long term change in neuronal excitability which increases sensation in the absence of stimuli, a process is known as neuronal remodelling. The broad range of chemicals that activate TRPA1 means that an initial chemical sensory exposure and subsequent tissue damage leads to sensitisation of TRPA1 channels through inflammatory pathways and finally prolonged hypersensitivity to multiple stimuli. TRPM8 can evoke a soothing and counter irritant in the nasal airway. Its role in modulating cough has not been clearly identified.

Airway afferent nerves

The first stage of reflexive cough occurs with stimulation and activation of the airway afferent nerve. Airway afferent nerves originate from the vagal nodose

19

(inferior) and jugular (superior) ganglia.[19] The fibres terminate in and under the airway epithelium[19] in the larynx and tracheobronchial tree but may also be present in the external auditory meatus, diaphragm, esophagus, pericardium, and stomach.

There are several different afferent nerve fibre types[5,18,19] and different ways of classifying them.[17] They can be described by function, origin, location in the airway, neurochemistry, electrophysiological properties or by reflexes that are evoked secondary to afferent activation.[17] These nerves respond to different types of stimuli and have different properties. The terminology used to describe airway afferent nerves in the literature can be confusing. In this text we use the terms *C-Fibre* to refer to nerves that respond to chemical stimulation, *cough receptor* to refer to nerves that respond to mechanical stimulation and *pulmonary stretch receptors* to refer to nerves that respond to constriction and inflation in the lower airways. However the term *cough receptor* has been used to refer to all airway afferent nerve types in the literature and the terms *mechanosensor* and *chemosensor* have also been substituted for cough receptors and C-Fibres respectively.

Airway afferent nerves are activated by mechanical or chemical stimuli.[19] Activation is mediated by the TRP channels and leads to depolarisation of the nerve cell. This depolarisation generates an action potential and transmits along the vagus nerve to the nucleus tractus solitarius where it is processed.[19,20] If the specificity and intensity of the afferent nerve signal is sufficient, the cough reflex will be triggered.[21]

C-Fibres

The first type of vagal afferent nerves are the C-Fibres. Neuronal pathways converge on TRPV1 and TRPA1 to increase C-Fibre excitability during inflammation.[18] C-Fibres are unmyelinated which allows for rapid access for chemical stimuli.[18] They are insensitive to mechanical stimulation but are sensitive to capsaicin, bradykinin, prostaglandin E2, ozone, nicotine, adenosine, and serotonin and are activated by stimulation of TRPV1 and TRPA1[13]. They have relatively slower conduction of < 2m/second.[13] Cell bodies of C-Fibres are in the jugular (superior) ganglia.[13] C-Fibres can sensitise cough but do not evoke cough.

Cough receptors

The second type of vagal afferent nerve is the cough receptor – a term with the potential to cause some confusion. Cough receptors are myelinated fibres.[13] In contrast to C-Fibres, cough receptors are mechanosensitive and relatively insensitive to capsaicin, methacholine, histamine, substance P, or neurokinin A13. As such they do not express ion channels TRPA1 or TRPV1[13] although chronic inflammation can lead to an expression of TRPV1 on myleinated fibres.[18] This may explain why patients with increased sensitivity to chemical stimuli also report increased sensitivity to innocuous mechanical stimuli such as swallowing hard food. The cell bodies of cough receptors are in the nodose (inferior) ganglion.[13] Cough receptors are found in the extrapulmonary airway including the larynx, trachea and mainstem bronchi.[13] They have more rapid conduction velocity of 5 m/second.[13] Termination occurs between the epithelial cell layers and smooth muscle.[13]

Pulmonary stretch receptors

The final group of afferent nerve types are the pulmonary stretch receptors. There are two types of pulmonary stretch receptor: the Rapidly Adapting Receptor (RAR) and the Slowly Adapting Receptor (SAR).[17] Pulmonary stretch receptors have a rapid conduction velocity of 15 m/second. They innervate the intrapulmonary airway and are activated by methacholine, histamine, substance P, adenosine, and Neurokinin A. This activation causes smooth muscle contraction and reduced lung compliance but does not directly cause cough. They are activated by sustained lung contraction. RARs are not sensitive to lung collapse or deflation. SARs are sensitive to mechanical forces on the lung during breathing. SARs are activated by sustained lung inflation and activation increases during inspiration. RARs are stimulated by bronchospasm. They are activated by negative intraluminal pressure such as during inspiratory effort against a closed glottis. The stretch receptors regulate respiratory rate, are sensitive to tussive stimuli, and regulate the duration and magnitude of inspiratory and expiratory phases of the cough.

Central projections

Cough involves both peripheral and central nervous systems. In the peripheral nervous system, cough is mediated by peripheral sensory nerves in the airways.[19] The mechanisms of chronic pain can be useful in understanding neural modula-

21

tion of the cough response. Inflammation typically occurs at the site of tissue injury and promotes healing. It results in pain which serves as a warning to protect the site from further injury. In addition to localised sensitisation, there is also a more central sensitisation due to the peripheral drive from the affected region to the brainstem. Thus, pain from inflammation can evolve into neuropathic pain.[22] This same process is thought to occur in chronic cough.

The afferent arm of the cough reflex is largely controlled by the vagus nerve.[23] The specific branches of the vagus nerve include the internal branch of the superior laryngeal nerve for the larynx, and the pulmonary branch for receptors lower down the tracheobronchial tree. The auricular branch of the vagus nerve innervates the external auditory meatus. Stimulation of the external auditory meatus can trigger cough in five percent of individuals.[13] The afferent arm of the cough reflex terminates on neurones near the nucleus tractus solitarius. There is a central processing of cough which integrates central and peripheral responses involving the nucleus ambiguus, retroambigulais, and phrenic nucleus. Cough may be generated via the reflex pathway when the cough stimulus has reached a reflex threshold in the brainstem.[16] There is synergistic interaction between C fibres and cough receptors which leads to enhanced cough responsiveness evoked by allergic inflammation, gastroesophageal reflux disease and upper airway diseases.[13] Increased responsiveness may reflect facilitatory central interactions of the esophagus or trigeminal pathways with cough processing in the brainstem. This process is summarised in Figure 2.1.

Although the vagus nerve has a significant role in cough, trigeminal afferent nerves also play a role in regulation of the cough reflex.[24] The trigeminal nerve contributes to the perception of airway irritation and the urge to cough. Stimulation of the trigeminal afferent cells in the nasal cavity can enhance the cough reflex[24] but does not necessarily lead to cough.[13,25] The increased cough response resulting from trigeminal stimulation requires integration of sensory information in the nucleus tractus solitarius. This process has a role in ensuring airway protection, for example triggering a defence mechanism when noxious substances enter the nasal cavity. There can be a sensitising effect of upper airway nerves which increases cough responsiveness and subsequently cough.[13] This hypothesis assumes that stimulation of the trigeminal nerve can promote cough by lowering the threshold of central cough pattern generator to subsequent input from the vagus nerve.[13] In other words, stimulation of the trigeminal

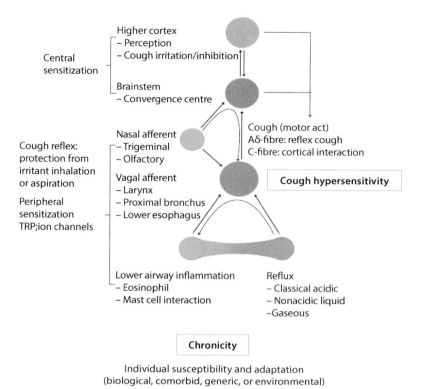

Figure 2.1: Adapted from Song.[19] Schematic presentation on the development of cough hypersensitivity. The key event may be the development of vagal neuronal hypersensitivity located in the airways. Commonly associated diseases such as rhinitis, eosinophilic airway inflammation, or classical acidic reflux may be triggers to lower thresholds for peripheral cough reflex activation. Nasal afferent stimulation may not directly initiate the cough reflex but may modulate the cough reflex either sensitising or desensitising, depending on the type of nasal stimulus. Gaseous reflux has been hypothesized to be a common factor to develop cough hypersensitivity. TRP = transient receptor potential.

nerve reduces the threshold of the central cough pattern generator to subsequent vagus nerve input so that innocuous stimuli can promote cough.[13]

Many patients with chronic refractory cough report that their cough is triggered by perfumes or scents. This observation may lead one to question the role of the olfactory nerve in the modulation of cough. The function of the olfactory nerve is to identify odour and enable smell,[26] however it merely has an indirect role in the modulation of cough. In contrast, direct stimulation of airway afferent nerves occurs via the trigeminal nerve for nasal stimulation, the glossopharyngeal nerve for pharyngeal sensation and the vagus nerve for laryngeal stimulation. Airborne pollution may involve both cognitive odour annoyance and irritant components. Odour concentration generally precedes sensory irritation and individuals are likely to report respiratory symptoms in response to odour but without reaching irritation and toxicity thresholds.[27]

Cortical control of cough

Although cough is reflexive, the cerebral cortex has a significant role in the modulation of cough. The cerebral cortex is responsible for the cognitive processes involved in cough[5] and is involved in planning, initiating and controlling motor output to the respiratory muscles during cough.[23] Cortical control is important for voluntary cough and for the decision to suppress a cough following an urge to cough.[23] The cerebral cortex also provides input during reflexive cough.

Initiation of the cough may be due to a sensation of irritation caused by physical or chemical stimuli, or the presence of inflammatory mediators that cause hypersensitivity of cough receptors during acute upper airway tract viral infections. Following the relay of information from the sensory afferents to the respiratory area of the brainstem, information is passed to the cerebral cortex where the sensation of irritation is mediated.[17,10] The patient's perception of the magnitude of the stimulus does not necessarily equate to the actual magnitude of the stimulus and can be affected by emotion, attention and alertness.[28] The cerebral cortex may initiate the cough response by acting centrally on the respiratory area of the brainstem, which allows the cough to be initiated at will and be voluntarily suppressed.

Functional magnetic resonance imaging (fMRI) studies (see Figure 2.2) have provided insights into the role of the cerebral cortex in modulating cough. There are also similarities in fMRI studies of the regions involved in cough and those involved in pain, dyspnea and esophageal distention.[23]

The areas involved in cough include the motor cortex, sensory motor cortex, supplementary motor area, and limbic system. The degree of cortical activation varies between brain regions. For example, activation of the anterior insular occurs in a stimulus dependent fashion. In contrast, activation of the primary sensory cortex occurs according to the individual's perception of the strength of the stimulus. The orbitofrontal cortex and cingulate cortex can influence an individual's affective response to airway irritation and thus influence their urge to cough.[23]

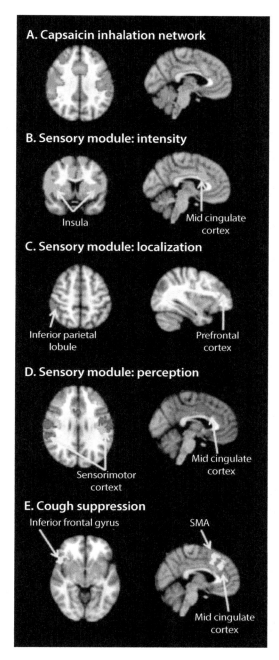

A. Capsaicin inhalation network

B. Sensory module: intensity

Insula   Mid cingulate cortex

C. Sensory module: localization

Inferior parietal lobule   Prefrontal cortex

D. Sensory module: perception

Sensorimotor cortext   Mid cingulate cortex

E. Cough suppression

Inferior frontal gyrus   SMA

Mid cingulate cortex

Figure 2.2: Functional brain maps of sensorimotor activations following capsaicin inhalation in humans. **(A)** Capsaicin inhalation is associated with the activation of a distributed network in the brain. Mazzone *et al.*[23] propose that this network is composed of several sub-circuits (modules) involved in sensory discrimination and motor control (panels B–E). Discrete regional responses incorporate modules that **(B)** encode stimulus intensity, **(C)** identify stimulus location, **(D)** determine perceptual experiences, and **(E)** can suppress evoked motor responses.

The urge to cough is encoded in several areas of the cerebral cortex. These areas include the primary sensory cortex which is mainly responsible for encoding the intensity of the urge to cough, the insula which encodes the magnitude of the incoming sensory input from the airway, and the pre-frontal and post parietal cortices which are responsible for attention and localisation of the site of irritation.[13]

There is different processing of both voluntary and reflexive coughing at the cortical and brainstem level. Voluntary cough involves the premotor and motor cortex, cerebellum, and corticospinal pathway.[13] Importantly, voluntary cough occurs without medullary input. The limbic and orbitofrontal cortex is involved in processing affective components such as unpleasantness.[13]

Voluntary cough suppression involves different regions of the brain than voluntary cough initiation. The specific regions involved in voluntary cough suppression are the anterior insula, supplementary motor area, motor cingulate cortex and right inferior frontal gyrus.[29] In contrast, placebo inhibition involves the dorsolateral prefrontal cortex which is the same area involved with placebo analgesia.[13]

Efferent pathway

The efferent pathway for the cough begins with motor information being processed in the cerebral cortex, cerebellum and the nucleus ambiguus.[30] The motor outputs send motor neurones to the inspiratory and expiratory muscles, larynx and bronchial tree[31] via descending efferent pathways. The efferent arm of the cough activates the recurrent laryngeal, phrenic, intercostal, and thoracoabdominal nerves.[32] An action potential is carried via the efferent nerves to the laryngeal and respiratory muscles[19] to produce a cough. Inspiratory and expiratory muscles are innervated by phrenic and spinal motor nerves by the nucleus retroambiualis while the laryngeal muscles are innervated by the recurrent laryngeal nerve via the nucleus ambiguus. The effector muscles are those involved in glottal closure, diaphragm relaxation, and thoracic and abdominal muscle contraction.

Summary

The anatomy and physiology of cough is complex and varies according to whether the cough is voluntary or reflexive. The Urge to Cough model is a clinically useful method of conceptualising and measuring the stages from the initial cough stimulus to the cough and consequences of the cough. The components of neurophysiological control of cough incorporate transient receptor potentials, afferent airway nerves, central projections and cortical control and can be modified in the development and treatment of chronic cough.

References

1. DelDonno M, Aversa C, Corsico R, *et al.* Efficacy and safety of moguisterine in comparison with dextromethorphan in patients with persistent cough. *Drug Investigation.* 1994;7(2):92–100.

2. Ferrari M, Oliveri D, Sembenini C, *et al.* Tussive effect of capsaicin in patients with gastroesophageal reflux without cough. *American Journal of Respiratory and Critical Care Medicine.* 1995;151:557–61.

3. Irwin R, Boulet L, Cloutier M, *et al.* Managing cough as a defence mechanism and as a symptom: A consensus report for the American College of Chest Physicians. *Chest.* 1998;114(2):133S (47).

4. Widdicome J. Neurophysiology of the cough reflex. *European Respiratory Journal.* 1995;8(7):1193–202.

5.   McGarvey L, McKeagney P, Polley L, *et al*. Are there clinical features of a sensitized cough reflex? *Pulmonary Pharmacology & Therapeutics*. 2009;22:59–64.

6.   Widdicome J, Fontana GA. Cough: what's in a name? *European Respiratory Journal*. 2006;28:10–15.

7.   Fontana GA. Before we get started: what is a cough? *Lung*. 2008;186(1):2.

8.   Vertigan A, Gibson P. Urge to cough and its application to the behavioural treatment of cough. *Bratislava Medical Journal*. 2011;3:102–8.

9.   Hilton E, Marsden P, Thurston A, *et al*. Clinical features of the urge-to-cough in patients with chronic cough. *Respiratory Medicine*. 2015;109(6):701–7.

10.   Davenport P. Urge to cough: what can it teach us about cough. *Lung*. 2008;186(S1):107–11.

11.   Davenport P, Sapienza C, Bolser D. Psychophysical assessment of the urge to cough. *European Respiratory Journal*. 2002;12:249–53.

12.   Farrer J, Keenan J, Levy P. Understanding the pathology and treatment if virus-induced cough. *Home Healthcare Consultant*. 2001;82(2):10–8.

13.   Canning BJ, Chang AB, Bolser DC, *et al*. Anatomy and neurophysiology of cough: Chest guideline and expert panel report. *Chest*. 2014;146(6):1633–48.

14.   Philp E. Chronic cough. *American Family Physician*. 1997;56(5):1395–404.

15.   Spinney L. Get it off your chest. *New Scientist*. 2002;November.

16.   Lee P, Cotterill-Jones C, Eccles R. Voluntary control of cough. *Pulmonary Pharmacology & Therapeutics*. 2002;15(3):317–20.

17.   Mazzone S. An overview of the sensory receptors regulating cough. *Cough*. 2005;1(2).

18.   Bessac B, Jordt S-E. Breathtaking TRP channels: trpa1 and TRPV1 in airway chemosensation and reflex control. *Physiology*. 2008;23:360–70.

19.   Song W-J, Chang Y-S, Morice A. Changing the paradigm for cough: does 'cough hypersensitivity' aid our understanding? *Asia Pacific Allergy*. 2013;4(1):3–13.

20.   Canning B. Cough Sensors I: Physiological and pharmacological properties of the afferent nerves regulating cough. In: Chung K, Widdicombe J (eds). *Handbook of Experimental Pharmacology*. Heidelberg, Berlin: Springer-Verlag; 2008.

21.   Chang AB. Cough, cough receptors, and asthma in children. *Pediatric Pulmonology*. 1999;28(1):59–70.

22.   Rahman W, Dickenson AH. Voltage gated sodium and calcium channel blockers for the treatment of chronic inflammatory pain. *Neuroscience Letters*. 2013;17(557):19–26.

23.   Mazzone S, McGovern AE, Yang S-K, *et al*. Sensorimotor circuitry involved in the higher brain control of coughing. *Cough*. 2013;9(7).

24.   Buday T, Brozmanova M, Biringerova Z, *et al*. Modulation of cough response by sensory inputs from the nose - role of trigeminal TRPA1 versus TRPM8 channels. *Cough*. 2012;8(11).

27

25. Plevkova J, Biringerova Z, Gavliakova S, *et al.* The role of nasal trigeminal nerves expressing TRP channels in modulation of cough threshold and urge to cough – possible clinical application. *Clinical and Translational Allergy*. 2013;Suppl 2(O17).

26. Gartner-Schmidt J, Rosen C, Radhakrishnan N, Ferguson B. Odor provocation test for laryngeal hypersensitivity. *Journal of Voice*. 2006;12(3):333–8.

27. Blanes-Vidal V, Balum J, Schwartz J, *et al.* Respiratory and sensory irritation symptoms among residents exposed to low-to-moderate air pollution from biodegradable wastes. *Journal of Exposure Science and Environmental Epidemiology*. 2014;24(4):388–97.

28. Mazzone SB, McLennan L, McGovern AE, *et al.* Representation of capscaisin evoked urge to cough in human brain using functional MRI. *American Journal of Respiratory and Critical Care Medicine*. 2007;176(4):327–32.

29. Leech J, Mazzone SB, Farrell MJ. Brain activity associated with placebo suppression of the urge-to-cough in humans. *American Journal of Respiratory and Critical Care Medicine*. 2013;188(9):1069–75.

30. Chu M, Lieser J, Sinacori J. Use of botulinum toxin type A for chronic cough: a neuropathic model. *Archives of Otolaryngology Head and Neck Surgery*. 2010;136(5):447–52.

31. French C, Irwin R, Curley F, Krikorian C. Impact of chronic cough on quality of life. *Archives of Internal Medicine*. 1998;158(15):1657–61.

32. Polverino M, Polverino F, Fasolino M, *et al.* Anatomy and neuro-pathophysiology of the cough reflex arc. *Multidiscip Resp Med*. 2012;7(1):5.

3

Medical conditions associated with chronic cough

Peter G. Gibson and Anne E. Vertigan

Chronic cough is associated with a wide range of seemingly unrelated medical conditions. However, recognition and treatment of these conditions forms a key part of the management of chronic cough. In this chapter, we review the medical conditions that have a recognised association with chronic cough, and present an approach to managing these issues.

What links these disorders to chronic cough?

The medical conditions associated with chronic cough are listed in Table 3.1. The link between these conditions and chronic cough is complex. Relevant issues are the anatomic reason for the association between the medical disorders and cough, whether the association is causal, why only some patients with the medical disorders develop chronic cough, and why a therapeutic response can be incomplete. The link between these disorders and chronic cough is best understood by understanding the innervation of the vagus nerve. The vagus nerve innervates many parts of the aero-digestive tract, and its name, meaning 'the wanderer' in Latin, reflects the wide array of sites innervated by this nerve. This has practical management implications since the assessment of chronic cough using the Anatomic Diagnostic Protocol[1] is based around the known sites of sensory innervation by the vagus nerve.

What remains to be determined?

Asthma, gastroesophageal reflux disease (GERD), and rhinosinusitis are the most common conditions associated with chronic cough, once serious lung disorders have been excluded.[1] Together, these three conditions are present in between 70% and 90% of patients with chronic cough. However, to add to the complexity, not all people with these disorders develop chronic cough, indicating that additional factors are required to cause chronic cough. At present, it is unclear why only some people with these conditions develop chronic cough.[2,3] It has been hypothesised that co-existing cough reflex hypersensitivity is present in the subset of patients with these medical conditions who develop chronic cough. In these cases it is more likely that GERD, asthma, and rhinosinusitis are acting as triggers in an already hypersensitive system.

| Gastroesophageal reflux disease |
| Rhinosinusitis |
| Asthma |
| Obstructive sleep apnoea |
| Eosinophilic bronchitis |
| ACE-inhibitor use |

Table 3.1: Medical conditions associated with chronic cough.

It is also unclear whether there is a causal relationship between these disorders and chronic cough. This is because not all of the criteria of causality have been demonstrated. For these conditions to be causal it would need to be proved that (1) there was a temporal association between the disease and cough, (2) that there was a dose relationship, and (3) treatment of the underlying disease relieved cough symptoms.[4] We know that this is not true in the majority of individuals. For example, although reflux of gastric acid is a potent trigger of cough, randomized trials of acid suppression do not clearly demonstrate resolution of cough.[5,6]

Medical treatment of cough is often aimed treating the associated medical condition, for example, gastroesophageal reflux disease or asthma. In many cases the treatment might be effective for the underlying condition but fail to be effective for cough. It is important to differentiate between cough that responds to treatment for these conditions and cough that does not respond. For example, an individual with symptoms of cough and gastroesophageal reflux may who is treated with antireflux medication may experience resolution of the reflux symptoms but not of the cough symptoms.

Gastroesophageal reflux

Reflux of stomach contents can be a normal physiological event, however frequent reflux can cause neural activation in either the distal esophagus or more proximally, and can also lead to acid-induced tissue damage and inflammation. Once this happens, the patient can develop symptoms of heartburn and reflux. This is a well described condition which responds well to lifestyle modification and acid suppression. A second situation occurs when the gastric reflux is associated with the development of symptoms that are not typical for reflux, termed 'atypical GERD'.[7] These symptoms include chest pain, chronic cough, dysphonia, globus, and orodental disease. The association between chronic cough and gastroesophageal reflux can be present as a part of GERD, or as an isolated symptom and part of the atypical presentation of GERD.

Gastroesophageal reflux disease

GERD can be classified by both the content of the reflux and the location of the reflux. In terms of location it can be broadly classified into distal reflux (reflux into the distal esophagus), laryngopharyngeal reflux without aspiration where there is laryngeal irritation by direct stimulation with gastric contents, and laryngopharyngeal reflux with aspiration into the respiratory tract where there is micro aspiration of gastric contents. Laryngopharyngeal reflux is often diagnosed based on laryngeal signs but these are not specific and may be the result of other pathophysiological mechanisms.[4] There is no gold standard for diagnosing laryngopharyngeal reflux.[8] Oesphagitis is uncommon in cough.

In terms of content, gastroesophageal reflux can also be classified as acidic, weakly acidic, non-acidic or gaseous. Cough symptoms in acid and non-acid reflux are very similar. It is argued that an incomplete response of chronic cough to acid suppression with proton pump inhibitor treatment can be due to non-acid reflux.[20]

Clinical tests for gastroesophageal reflux

A number of clinical tests can be used to diagnose gastroesophageal reflux. Twenty four hour ambulatory esophageal pH monitoring has long been considered the gold standard for diagnosing reflux. In this test a probe is placed into the esophagus and detects acid levels over a 24-hour period. The clinical utility of pH monitoring in the management of chronic cough has been questioned as results do not predict an individual's response of cough to anti-reflux therapy[9,10] and it does not detect non-acid reflux.[10] Other limitations are that there is no difference in acid exposure times between individuals who respond and those who fail to respond to anti-reflux therapy, and pH monitoring has a poor positive predictive value for response to anti-reflux medication in chronic cough.[11] These discrepancies may be explained by the requirement for additional factors in addition to acid reflux in causing chronic cough, or by the proposal that patients with chronic cough due to acid reflux have an increased sensitivity to normal amounts of acid exposure. Both of these explanations are consistent with the presence of cough reflex hypersensitivity as an essential component in GERD associated cough.

Newer techniques such as esophageal impedance pH monitoring[12] are gaining popularity in the research field. The probes used during this test are able to differentiate between solid, liquid and gaseous esophageal contents. These techniques therefore have the advantage of being able to diagnose non-acid reflux. However this testing is not routinely available outside specialist centres and is very expensive.[4] It is difficult to measure acid levels in the pharynx as the upper probe tends to dry out in the pharynx.[4]

There is little clinical utility of gastroscopy and barium swallow examination in the diagnosis of gastroesophageal reflux as a cause of cough. In practice gastroesophageal reflux is often diagnosed based on self-reported symptoms and response to reflux treatment.

Reflux treatment

Treatment options for GERD include behavioural strategies, pharmaceutical treatment or surgery. When evaluating the results of reflux treatment for an individual it is essential to differentiate between cough that responds to reflux treatment and cough that remains refractory to reflux treatment. Effective treatment of reflux can relieve cough symptoms in some patients[13] but is not universally effective.

Lifestyle modification for reflux

Lifestyle modification for reflux includes diet modifications, lifestyle changes, weight loss, raising the head of the bed when sleeping, and gum chewing.[14,15]

Proton pump inhibitors

Proton pump inhibitors are commonly used in the treatment of gastroesophageal reflux and are effective in treating gastroesophageal symptoms. The mechanism of action is to inhibit acid production rather than suppress reflux episodes. In other words a patient taking proton pump inhibitors may still have reflux episodes but the content of the reflux will be less acidic.

Early literature suggested that proton pump inhibitor medication for cough was effective in treating the condition. However several authors have now questioned the effectiveness of the medication. In a meta-analysis of studies on GERD and cough, Chang *et al.*[5] reported that the treatment effect of proton pump inhibitors on cough in randomised trials was smaller than the effects reported in early non-randomised trials and that the effect of proton pump inhibitor medication on cough associated with GERD is less convincing than suggested by consensus guidelines for the management of cough. Proton pump inhibitors do not result in improved cough severity and are not significantly better than placebo in treating cough due to reflux. Laryngopharyngeal reflux symptoms resolve more slowly than gastroesophageal symptoms following proton pump inhibitor treatment.[16]

Fundoplication

Fundoplication involves wrapping the superior portion of the stomach around the distal esophagus in order to prevent stomach contents refluxing into the esophagus. Surgical options are usually a last resort.[17] There have been no controlled studies of the effects of fundoplication on cough[6] although some reports suggest that up to 60% of patients may improve. Our clinical experience has found that while fundoplication is beneficial in controlling reflux it is not beneficial in relieving cough symptoms.

Reflux – cough relationship

Determining whether or not reflux is a cause of cough can be problematic and controversial. Gastroesophageal reflux has been correlated with cough[18] however does not universally result in chronic cough or paradoxical vocal fold movement[3] and a significant proportion of persons with GERD have no upper airway symptoms.[19] Reflux can occur in the normal population and can be triggered by cough episodes themselves.[20–22] Some patients only develop reflux symptoms after onset of the cough suggesting that cough can initiate the cough-reflux self-

33

perpetuating cycle.[22] In a study designed to examine the temporal relationship between chronic cough and reflux, Laukka *et al.*[23] found that more episodes of cough were not associated with reflux episodes and that cough was more likely to precede than to follow a reflux episode. Only a small number of patients have reflux events that are causally related to the cough. Smith[20] demonstrated that only a small number of cough episodes were temporally related to reflux episodes. Therefore, in these patients a reduction is unlikely to lead to a reduction in cough. But 48% of patients with chronic cough have a temporal association between reflux and cough. Smith found that 44% of cough episodes followed a reflux event whereas 56% of cough episodes were followed by a reflux event. Reflux can exist in patients with cough from other conditions.[10] Chang *et al.*[5] concluded that GERD and cough are common and often coincide but are not necessarily causal.

The physiology of the reflux - cough relationship can occur in two ways.[4] The first mechanism is by stimulation of the vagal esophageal bronchial reflex by intraoesophageal reflux. The stimulation of this reflex occurs due to hypersensitivity. However, intraoesophageal acid infusion only increases sensitivity of the cough reflex in patients who have both reflux and airway disease. Therefore, cough reflex sensitivity does not increase in patients with only airway disease or with only reflux disease. Reflux in the distal esophagus is caused by a neuronal mechanism.

The second mechanism in the reflux – cough relationship is regurgitation where the cough is a symptom of laryngopharyngeal reflux or microaspiration. Laryngopharyngeal reflux is diagnosed by thickening oedema and erythema in the laryngeal region. It is tempting to suggest that laryngopharyngeal reflux is the cause for cough in many patients. Laryngopharyngeal reflux is frequently discussed in the otolaryngology literature and can be considered a cause of coughing and throat clearing. In contrast, Birring[10] suggests that laryngopharyngeal reflux is less strongly recognised by respiratory physicians. The temporal association between laryngopharyngeal reflux and cough has not been demonstrated.[4] Refluxate reaches the larynx in patients with chronic cough with the same frequency as controls. This finding suggests that the presence of refluxate in the pharynx is not causative to the cough.

Microaspiration has also been argued as a cause for chronic cough. However bronchoalveolar lavage samples taken from patients with chronic cough are no different from those in healthy controls.[4] Aspiration and laryngopharyngeal reflux are thought to be less likely in chronic cough because pepsin and bile acid levels are not significantly different between patients with chronic cough and controls. There is limited difference in reflux occurring in healthy individuals and that occurring in patients with chronic cough. For example, episodes of reflux in patients with chronic cough are no different from healthy controls.[24] Smith reported that patients with chronic cough do not have excessive reflux.[4] The number and acidity of intraesophageal reflux is the same between patients with chronic cough and healthy controls. These findings support the hypothesis that patients with chronic cough have increased sensitivity to normal reflux events.

Effect of proton pump inhibitors on cough

Proton pump inhibitor medication has frequency been discussed as a treatment for chronic cough due to reflux. Proton pump inhibitors are more effective in patients with demonstrated reflux than in those with unexplained cough.[4] However, proton pump inhibitors are not effective in a substantial number of patients with reflux related cough.[4] Furthermore, Smith reported that no studies have found that reducing reflux events reduces cough.[4] These arguments suggest that the relationship between reflux and cough is an association rather than causal.[4]

The failure of proton pump inhibitors to effectively treat cough suggests that another mechanism may be occurring. Birring[24] proposed that non-acid reflux might be an important mechanism as proton pump inhibitors remove the acid from reflux but do not stop the reflux events from occurring. Factors other than acid such as pepsin might be involved in reflux related cough,[22,25] which would explain why cough can persist despite maximal reflux treatment.[26,27]

Rhinosinusitis

Rhinosinusitis is frequently associated with chronic cough.[18] Chronic inflammation of the nose and/or sinuses can stimulate pharyngeal and laryngeal irritant receptors,[28] and has also been associated with PVFM.[29]

The American College of Chest Physicians adopted the term 'Upper Airway Cough Syndrome' to refer to cough due to rhinosinusitis. This term replaced the previous term of chronic cough due to post nasal drip syndrome. Rhinosinusitis is the term recognised and used by otolaryngologists. Due to the potential for confusion between the terms 'upper airway cough syndrome' and 'paradoxical vocal fold movement', the term rhinosinusitis will be used throughout this book.

Signs and symptoms of rhinosinusitis include facial pain or pressure, nasal obstruction, nasal or postnasal discharge or purulence and hyposmia.[30] Rhinosinusitis can be acute or chronic. Chronic rhinosinusitis has several different causes including allergic rhinitis, perennial non-allergic rhinitis, vasomotor rhinitis post infectious rhinitis, chronic (bacterial) rhinosinusitis, allergic fungal rhinosinusitis, and non-allergic rhinitis due to medication abuse, environmental irritants and pregnancy.[31] Signs of allergic rhinitis include nasal itching, nasal blockage, nasal discharge, conjunctivitis and nocturnal snoring. Relevant allergenic triggers can be identified by measuring allergen-specific IgE levels using skin prick testing or radioallergosorbent testing.

Viral infection and allergen induced rhinitis are associated with inflammation of the paranasal sinuses and this is the likely common factor that triggers cough. Post nasal drip involves a sensation of secretions at back of nose causing frequent throat clearing and could be considered a symptom of hypersensitivity.[32] Experimental studies suggest that in healthy people mechanical stimulation of cough receptors by post-nasal drip does not occur. However in chronic rhinosinusitis it is unclear whether post nasal discharge stimulates cough receptors in the pharynx or whether mucus or inflammation stimulate cough receptors in the paranasal sinuses.[33]

PVFM has also been associated with sinusitis. Rolla *et al.*[34] found a high prevalence of extrathoracic airway hyperresponsiveness in people with chronic cough associated with chronic sinusitis. Rolla *et al.* studied the relationship between sinusitis, airway dysfunction and morphologic changes in the pharyngeal mucosa, and concluded that sinusitis causes pharyngeal damage that subsequently led to extrathoracic airway hyperresponsiveness. Patients with extrathoracic airway hyperresponsiveness had significantly thinner pharyngeal epithelium. Histamine inhalation challenge performed during an exacerbation of chronic sinusitis showed an early marked decrease in maximal inspiratory flows consistent with a constrictive response at the pharyngolaryngeal level. Eighty percent of patients with confirmed extrathoracic airway hyperresponsiveness in this study also reported a cough. Rolla *et al.* concluded that sinusitis led to pharyngeal damage that subsequently led to extrathoracic airway hyperresponsiveness. Changes in olfaction or trigeminal receptors may be an additional mechanism by which non-allergic rhinitis triggers PVFM.[8]

In adults, chronic rhinosinusitis as a cause of chronic cough is suggested by nasal or upper airway symptoms of more than 12 weeks' duration and at least two of the following symptoms or signs: anterior and/or posterior mucopurulent drainage, nasal obstruction, facial pressure, pain or fullness.[35] Investigation can involve a CT scan of the sinuses. This is indicated when the diagnosis is uncertain, the patient is not responding to medical treatment as expected, or surgery is planned or being considered.

Management includes medical and surgical management of sinus disease and allergy including topical nasal corticosteroids, antihistamines, antibiotics and allergen management.[35] Oral antibiotic therapy for between three weeks and three months is used for purulent chronic rhinosinusitis. Additional treatment for allergic rhinitis includes restriction to likely exposures, exclusion of specific allergens,[35] and desensitization with allergen immunotherapy.

It is important to differentiate between cough that responds to treatment for rhinosinusitis and cough that persists despite this treatment. In fact, many cases of cough associated with rhinosinisitis remain refractory to this treatment. Patients may have clear sinus but still have post nasal discharge and rhinitis.

Asthma

Asthma a disease of the lower airways (bronchi) resulting in spasm of the bronchi leading to symptoms of wheeze, shortness of breath and cough. The underlying mechanisms involve inflammation and increased responsiveness of the airways to triggers. Asthma is frequently associated with chronic cough and PVFM. Cough variant asthma is a variation of asthma primarily characterised by cough, rather than wheeze or shortness of breath.

A number of methods are used to diagnose asthma. In clinical practice, asthma is often diagnosed by symptoms, spirometry and response to bronchodilators. If spirometry is normal, then bronchial provocation testing can be used to diagnose asthma. Provocation testing is described in more detail in Chapter 4. In difficult to manage asthma, additional assessment including measurement of airway inflammation can be helpful. This testing will determine whether there are increased eosinophils or neutrophils present in the sample.

Treatment of asthma involves beta-2agonists which are used as bronchodilators, and inhaled corticosteroids to reduce airway inflammation. This can lead to resolution of cough in a number of patients. Despite this, cough can persist despite optimal asthma treatment. Similar to GERD and rhinitis, the clinician needs to differentiate between cough that responds to treatment for asthma, and cough that persists despite asthma treatment. It is essential that associated asthma is managed by a respiratory physician prior to referral to speech pathology.

ACE Inhibitors

Angiotensin converting enzyme (ACE) inhibitors are a class of medication used to treat hypertension. ACE inhibitors increase cough reflex sensitivity and, thus, have been associated with chronic cough. ACE inhibitors may also increase cough sensitivity in cough due to other causes. For example, ACE inhibitors may increase cough reflex sensitivity in patients with cough resulting from asthma or gastroesophageal reflux disease. The inhibition of ACE leads to increased levels of bradykinin, which is a mediator that activates airway sensory nerves to cause cough.

It is important to note that there does not need to be a temporal association between the onset of cough and commencing ACE inhibitors. Many patients may have been taking ACE inhibitors for years before the onset of cough. These patients may have increased cough reflex sensitivity as a result of the ACE inhibitor and the onset of new disease acts as a trigger to increase cough frequency.

Treatment of cough associated with ACE inhibitor use involves a trial of withdrawing the ACE inhibitor. This trial needs to be done with careful medical management and it is not the role of the speech pathologist to recommend this treatment. In some cases, patients taking ACE inhibitors may be referred to speech pathology and the speech pathologist may need to check whether a trial of withdrawing the ACE inhibitor has been considered by the referring physician. However this should be discussed directly with the referring physician. Some patients may misinterpret the suggestion that you are going to check with the physician with advice to stop the ACE inhibitor.

Obstructive sleep apnoea

Obstructive sleep apnoea is one of the more recently recognised diseases associated with chronic cough.[36] It is a condition characterised by repetitive episodes of upper airway occlusion during sleep, associated with sleep fragmentation, and daytime hypersomnolence.[37]

Obstructive sleep apnoea is treated with a Continuous Positive Airway Pressure (CPAP) which is worn over the nose and/or mouth at night. Birring[24] claimed that CPAP leads to a significant reduction in cough or in some cases a resolution in cough. The mechanism of improvement in cough is thought to occur through two processes. The first is an increase in transdiaphragmatic pressure in apnoea, leading to reduced lower esophageal pressure. The second mechanism is that cough is the result of upper airway inflammation associated with epithelial injury associated with snoring apnoea.

Eosinophilic bronchitis

Eosinophilic bronchitis is a feature of many respiratory diseases and is characterised by increased eosinophils in the sputum.[38] Gibson[39] found that eosinophilic bronchitis is a cause of chronic cough and that successful treatment of the condition reduces cough severity. Treatment involves inhaled and occasionally oral corticosteroids.

Psychological conditions

A psychological basis for chronic cough has been implicated in the literature. Assertions regarding a psychological basis for chronic cough must be interpreted carefully. While psychological considerations cannot be denied, there is a danger of using psychological and psychiatric labels simply because an organic cause cannot be identified. Although psychological issues may coexist with chronic cough, the nature of causality in this relationship has not been confirmed and the co-existence of psychological issues should not be over-interpreted as being causal. It is suggested therefore that psychogenic labels should not be used simply because a medical cause cannot be found, but rather once psychiatric issues have been systematically investigated and diagnosed, and found to be the cause of the symptoms.

There is no empirical evidence linking psychogenic cough with underlying psychic conflict, or with more serious psychopathology.[40] Chronic cough itself may lead to or exacerbate psychological symptoms and have negative emotional side effects.[41]

A number of studies have investigated psychological issues in patients with chronic cough. Carney *et al.*[3] examined psychiatric symptomatology in subjects with chronic cough using a validated psychological profile questionnaire, the Symptom Checklist-90 item revised. The 90 items in the scale were clustered into nine clinical axes of psychopathology, including somatization, obsessive-compulsive, interpersonal sensitivity, depression, anxiety, hostility, phobic anxiety, paranoid ideation and psychosis. Patients with chronic cough had significantly higher scores in the somatisation and hostility domains compared with controls, however there were no significant differences in scores between subjects and controls in the other psychological domains. Carney *et al.* questioned whether psychiatric disease may predispose patients to develop chronic cough, or whether chronic cough may cause psychiatric symptoms. Regardless of the actual cause, chronic cough could provide secondary gain by freeing sufferers from obligations perceived as threatening, or by securing special consideration. In contrast, Lokshin *et al.*[42] found no somatisation or emotional disorders in their patients with habitual cough.

McGarvey[43] found increased anxiety and depression scores on the Hospital Anxiety and Depression Scale (HADS)[44] of 33% and 16%, respectively, of patients with chronic cough. These levels were similar to those found in other respiratory diagnoses. Trait anxiety, i.e. underlying tendency to anxiety, on the State Trait Anxiety Inventory: was moderately high in 44% of patients with idiopathic cough, and in 4% of patients with treated cough. State anxiety, i.e. how anxious the individual currently is, was low in 72% of patients and moderate in 28% of patients. The Crown Crisp Experiential Index scores were increased compared with published norms, but lower than for psychiatric outpatient populations. Another study[45] demonstrated mean anxiety and depression scores to be within the normal range on the HADS, although up to 50% of patients with PVFM, and 33% of patients with chronic cough had anxiety scores in the *possible* or *probable* range.

These studies challenge the label of psychogenic cough for cough that is refractory to medical treatment, as a substantial proportion of patients with chronic cough and PVFM have normal anxiety and depression scores.

Dicpinigaitis *et al.*[46] found that 53% of their patients with chronic cough had a positive score on the Centre for Epidemiologic Studies Depression Scale. There was an improvement in both subjective cough scores and depression scores three months following medical treatment for the cough. No antidepressant medication was used in any of the patients.

Chronic cough has been conceptualised in terms of classical conditioning whereby breathing in air subsequently developed into a nervous habit.[47] This assertion has been supported by experiments with classical conditioning in guinea pigs, whereby associative learning enhanced the cough response.[48]

Psychological issues have been found to exacerbate symptoms in cough with known etiologies such as asthma whereby people with asthma coughed more often in situations that they had learned to associate with asthma rather than in one unrelated to asthma.[49] Mild levels of psychiatric symptoms such as anxiety have been associated with respiratory disorders such as asthma.

While psychiatric issues might contribute to respiratory symptoms such as cough, it is also possible for respiratory symptoms to contribute to psychological issues. For example, there may be a valid physiological explanation for feelings of anxiety to occur in chronic cough associated with PVFM. Many patients with cough associated with PVFM report a sensation of being choked during an episode of PVFM, causing some to fear that they will die during a dyspnoeic episode.[50,51] Wamboldt and Wamboldt[52] discussed the concept of a suffocation alarm and claimed that PVFM pathophysiology is due to hyperactivity of this alarm.

Psychological issues could also arise as a result of the side effects of chronic cough. There are numerous physical, social and emotional side effects to chronic cough. These side effects, including avoidance of activities, difficulty with interpersonal relationships, stress urinary incontinence and avoidance of talking, might have an impact on psychological health.[29,41]

Persisting symptoms may act as a stressor in patients with chronic cough. Lack of a firm diagnosis for chronic refractory cough can lead to psychological distress in some patients. The management of chronic refractory cough in primary care is variable, and patients may undergo extended series of investigations and treatment trials in attempt to diagnose and manage the symptoms. The lack of a firm diagnosis for respiratory symptoms in disorders can act as a stressor in itself.[53] In a series of focus groups, Ringsberg *et al.*[53] found that patients with cough reflex hypersensitivity and PVFM-like symptoms were more psychologically distressed, had more problems with their families and social lives, and sought more frequent medical care compared with a control group of patients with confirmed asthma.

The terms 'Psychogenic Cough' and 'Habit Cough' have been used to describe cough that has no obvious medical etiology, is refractory to medical management and considered to have a psychiatric or psychological basis.[1] The latest American Cough Guidelines have replaced the term 'Psychogenic Cough' with the term 'Somatic Cough Syndrome'.[54] However there is limited diagnostic criteria for psychogenic cough in the literature.[55] Information about diagnosis and treatment of psychogenic and habit cough are limited to small case series and expert opinion only. They appear to occur more frequently in children than adults. The classic description of psychogenic cough was of a barking, honking quality and that it was absent at night. However, more recent authors have found that cough due to organic disease can be absent at night and that a barking, honking quality can be present in other diseases.

Criticisms can be made regarding the conceptualisation and description of psychogenic cough reported in the literature. Several authors have warned that poor response to treatment for chronic cough could lead to the mistaken belief that the cough is functional or psychogenic, particularly when cause of the cough had not been appropriately investigated.[25,27] Kardos[56] suggested that a diagnosis of psychogenic cough should not coincide with hypersensitivity of the cough reflex. Yet many studies attributing cough to psychological causes have failed to consider cough reflex hypersensitivity or extrathoracic airway hyperresponsiveness, which sheds doubt on the validity of the psychogenic diagnosis.

The level of evidence for the diagnosis and management of psychogenic cough is based on expert opinion only.[55,57] Diagnostic criteria for psychogenic cough have been described, but have not been systematically assessed in a controlled setting.[57]

The term psychogenic cough implies that the cough is an expression of an underlying, usually unconscious conflict.[52,58] Milgrom *et al.*[58] stated that wholly psychogenic cough is rare but that psychological factors may affect the progression of symptoms. The definition and diagnostic criteria for psychogenic cough is unclear and has not been empirically confirmed in the literature. There have been no randomised controlled trials and in many studies the diagnosis of psychogenic cough has been made in the absence of a psychiatric assessment.

We argue that the label of psychogenic cough or somatic cough syndrome should not be used just because a cause for the cough cannot be found. Secondly, we argue that these labels should not be used just because an individual presents with an associated psychiatric condition. We know that some psychiatric disorders are a result rather than a cause of cough, and resolve once the cough is successfully treated.

Post viral cough

Cough is a common symptom associated with upper respiratory tract infection[59] and viral upper respiratory tract infection is a predominant trigger of coughing attacks in both acute and chronic cough.[60] There is evidence that post viral illness may cause hyperresponsiveness that subsequently manifests as chronic cough or PVFM. Cough reflex sensitivity increases following upper respiratory tract infection and usually returns to normal following resolution of the infection.[61] However, in some individuals cough reflex sensitivity remains elevated even after resolution of the infection. The pathogenesis of post viral cough could be due to airway inflammation with or without transient airway hyperresponsiveness.[60]

While post viral infection is not frequently listed in algorithms for the treatment of chronic cough, it could be an unrecognised contributing factor. Upper respiratory tract infection is related to increased cough reflex sensitivity. Anecdotally, a significant proportion of patients presenting to speech pathologists for management of chronic cough and hyperfunctional voice disorders report that the onset of symptoms coincided with upper respiratory tract infection.[62] The onset of cough in most patients with chronic cough is temporally associated with an upper respiratory tract infection.[63]

Serious medical conditions

Chronic cough can be associated with serious medical conditions (Table 3.2). It is essential that these conditions are identified and managed prior to referral for speech pathology treatment. In practice, it is unlikely that speech pathologists will encounter patients with cough caused by these serious medical condi-

Medical condition	Associated signs and symptoms
Neoplasm of larynx, bronchi, or lung	Haemoptysis
Cardiac failure	Dysphagia[64]
Tuberculosis[67]	Moderate–severe dysphonia
Pneumonia	Substantial sputum production
Interstitial lung disease	Prominent dyspnea
Lung abscess	Systemic symptoms e.g. fever or weight loss
Pulmonary infarction	Smoking
Extrinsic compression of trachea or	
bronchus e.g. from aortic aneurysm	

Table 3.2: Serious medical conditions associated with cough.

tions, because they will be managed according to a different treatment pathway. Nevertheless, it is important for the speech pathologist to be aware of these potentially serious medical conditions.

Other causes of cough

Other causes of chronic cough include smoking, lung pathology, protracted bacterial bronchitis,[35] chronic bronchitis, chronic obstructive pulmonary disease bronchiectasis, post viral infection, inhaled foreign bodies,[66] cystic fibrosis, parenchymal lung disease, irritant lesions in the external auditory meatus (Arnold's nerve), sarcoidosis, atopic cough, eosinophilic bronchitis,[27] familial sensory neuropathy of the superior and recurrent laryngeal nerves,[67] chronic tonsillar enlargement,[68] use of medications such as Angiotensin Conversion Enzyme inhibitors[1] or B-blockers. Several of these causes have not been investigated in large-scale studies and are yet to be incorporated into the routine protocols for management of chronic cough. It is beyond the scope of this book to discuss these issues in more detail.

An approach to the medical management of chronic cough

Several approaches have been recommended for the medical assessment of chronic cough. These can be based around identifying significant diseases, or the known associations of chronic cough, or the conditions most likely to be successfully treated. The approach described below uses elements of each of these approaches, and is based on the Australian cough guidelines (CICADA).[35]

The assessment revolves around determining:

1. Could the chronic cough be due to a serious underlying disease? (Table 3.2)
2. What are the most likely diagnoses to be present in a patient with chronic cough?
3. What conditions respond well to treatment?
4. What conditions should not be missed?

Could the chronic cough be due to a serious underlying disease?

This assessment is described above – see Table 3.2. It is essential that a serious underlying disease be identified and managed before undertaking speech pathology treatment for chronic cough. This process requires a medical history and examination, chest radiograph, spirometry, and targeted investigations as required.

What are the most likely diagnoses to be present in a patient with chronic cough?

This refers to a probability based diagnosis. If a clinical assessment, chest radiograph and spirometry are normal, then the most likely diseases associated with chronic cough are asthma, rhinosinusitis, GERD, and ACE-I use.

What conditions respond well to treatment?

Some conditions associated with chronic cough respond very well to treatment, and so it is important to recognise these. These conditions are protracted bacterial bronchitis, asthma, GERD, obstructive sleep apnea, eosinophilic bronchitis, and ACE-I use.

Centrally acting neuromodulators

Centrally acting neuromodulators such as gabapentin and pregabalin have been investigated in chronic cough and have an important role to play in reducing central sensitisation in chronic cough. These medications are typically used once cough is deemed refractory to medical treatment, however the timing of these and speech pathology treatment may vary according to patient and clinician preference. A double blind placebo controlled trial showed that gabapentin was effective in reducing cough frequency, cough quality of life, and cough severity.[69] When combined with speech pathology intervention, pregabalin reduces cough quality of life and cough severity more than speech pathology intervention alone.[70] Centrally acting neuromodulators, in contrast with speech pathology treatment, do not reduce cough reflex sensitivity. Furthermore, the treatment effect is not sustained once the medication is withdrawn. These medications can be limited by side effects which are managed by dose reduction.

Summary

A number of medical conditions are associated with chronic cough. The mechanisms linking these disorders to chronic cough are based around common vagal innervation. The medical assessment of chronic cough is an important precursor to speech pathology treatment. The purpose is to identify serious diseases causing cough, and to identify and treat remediable causes. A structured assessment can be performed to achieve these aims. If the cough persists after this assessment, then additional assessment and treatment is appropriate as described in the other chapters in this book.

References

1. Irwin R, Boulet L, Cloutier M, *et al.* Managing cough as a defence mechanism and as a symptom: A consensus report for the American College of Chest Physicians. *Chest.* 1998;114(2):133S (47).

2. Song W-J, Chang Y-S, Morice A. Changing the paradigm for cough: does 'cough hypersensitivity' aid our understanding? *Asia Pacific Allergy.* 2013;4(1):3–13.

3. Carney I, Gibson P, Murree-Allen K, *et al.* A systematic evaluation of mechanisms in chronic cough. *American Journal of Respiratory and Critical Care Medicine.* 1997;156(1):211–6.

4. Kahrilas P, Smith J, Dicpinigaitis P. A causal relationship between cough and gastroesophageal reflux disease (GERD) has been established: A pro/con debate. *Lung.* 2014;192(1):39–46.

5. Chang A, Lasserson T, Kiljander T, *et al.* Systematic review and meta-analysis of randomised controlled trials of gastro-oesophageal reflux interventions for chronic cough associated with gastro-oesophageal reflux. *British Medical Journal.* 2006;332(7532):11–7.

6. Chang A, Lasserson T, Gaffney J, *et al.* Gastro-oesophageal reflux treatment for prolonged non-specific cough in children and adults. *Cochrane Database of systematic Reviews.* 2011;1.

7. Abdul-Hussein M, Freeman J, Castell DO. Cough and throat clearing: atypical GERD symptoms or Not GERD at all? *Journal of Clinical Gastroenterology.* 2015;18:18.

8. Kenn K, Balkissoon R. Vocal cord dysfunction: what do we know? *European Respiratory Journal.* 2011;37:194–200.

9. McGarvey L. Clinical assessment of cough. In: Chung K, Widdicome J, Boushey H (eds). *Cough: Causes, Mechanisms and Therapy.* Melbourne: Blackwell Publishing; 2003.

10. Birring S. Controversies in the evaluation and management of chronic cough. *American Journal of Respiratory & Critical Care Medicine.* 2011;183(6):708–15.

11. Patterson R, Johnston B, MacMahon J, *et al.* Oesophageal pH monitoring is of limited value in the diagnosis of 'reflux-cough'. *European Respiratory Journal.* 2004;24:724–7.

12. Ribo P, Pacheco A, Arrieta P, *et al.* Gastroesophageal reflux as a cause of chronic cough, severe asthma, and migrtory pulmonary infiltrates. *Respirology Case Reports.* 2014;2(1):1–3.

13. Irwin RS. Chronic cough due to gastroesophageal reflux disease: ACCP evidence based clinical practice guidelines. *Chest.* 2006;129:80S–94S.

14. Smith J, Morjaria J, Morice A. Dietary intervention in the treatment of patients with cough and symptoms suggestive of airways reflux as determined by Hull airways Reflux Questionnaire. *Cough.* 2013;9(1):27.

15. Smoak B, Koufman J. Effects of gum chewing on pharyngeal and oesophageal pH. *Annals of Otology, Rhinology & Laryngology*. 2001;110(12):1117–9.

16. Oridate N, Takeda H, Asaka M, *et al*. Acid-suppression therapy offers varied laryngopharyngeal and esophageal symptom relief in laryngopharyngeal reflux patients. *Digestive Diseases & Sciences*. 2008;53(8):2033–8.

17. Kahrilas P. Maximizing outcome of extraesophageal reflux disease. *American Journal of Managed Care*. 2000;16(16Suppl):876–82.

18. Ludviksdottir D, Bjorusson E, Janson C, Boman G. Habitual coughing and its associations with asthma, anxiety and gastroesophageal reflux. *Chest*. 1996;109:1262–8.

19. Theodoropoulos DS, Ledford DK, Lockey RF, *et al*. Prevalence of upper respiratory symptoms in patients with symptomatic gastroesophageal reflux disease. *American Journal of Critical Care Medicine*. 2001;164:72–6.

20. Smith J, Decalmer S, Kelsall A, *et al*. Acoustic cough-reflux associations in chronic cough: potential triggers and mechanisms. *Gastroenterology*. 2010;139:754–2.

21. Chang A. Causes, assessment and measurement of cough in children. In: Chung K, Widdicome J, Boushey H (eds). *Cough: Causes, Mechanisms and Therapy*. Melbourne: Blackwell Publishing; 2003.

22. Ing A. Cough and gastroesophageal reflux. In: Chung K, Widdicome J, Boushey H (eds). *Cough: Causes, Mechanisms and Therapy*. Melbourne: Blackwell Publishing; 2003.

23. Laukka M, Cameron A, Schei A. Gastroesophageal reflux and chronic cough: Which comes first? *Journal of Clinical Gastroenterology*. 1994;19(2):100–4.

24. Birring S. New concepts in the management of chronic cough. *Pulmonary Pharmacology & Therapeutics*. 2011;24(3):334–8.

25. Chung K. The clinical and pathophysiological challenge of cough. In: Chung K, Widdicome J, Boushey H (eds). *Cough: Causes, Mechanisms and Therapy*. Melbourne: Blackwell Publishing; 2003.

26. Murry T, Tabaee A, Aviv J. Respiratory retraining of refractory cough and laryngopharyngeal reflux in patients with paradoxical vocal fold movement disorder. *The Laryngoscope*. 2004;114(8):1341–5.

27. McGarvey L, Forsythe P, Heaney L, *et al*. Idiopathic chronic cough: A real disease or a failure of diagnosis. *Cough*. 2005;1(9).

28. Newman K, Milgrom H. Chronic cough: A step by step diagnostic workup. *Consultant*. 1995;35(10):1535–7.

29. Brugman S. What's this thing called vocal cord dysfunction? *Primary and Critical Care Update*. 2006;20(26).

30. Osguthorpe D. Adult rhinosinusitis: diagnosis and management. *American Family Physician*. 2001. p. 69–77.

31. Palombini B, Araujo E. Cough in postnasal drip, rhinits and rhonosinusitis. In: Chung K, Widdicome J, Boushey H (eds). *Cough: Causes, Mechanisms and Therapy*. Melbourne: Blackwell Publishing; 2003.

32. Chung K. Chronic 'cough hypersensitivity syndrome': a more precise label for chronic cough. *Pulmonary Pharmacology & Therapeutics*. 2011;24(3):267–71.

33. Braman S, Corrao W. Chronic cough: Diagnosis and treatment. *Primary Care*. 1985;12(2):217–25.

34. Rolla G, Colagrande P, Scappaticci E, *et al*. Damage of the pharyngeal mucosa and hyperresponsiveness of airway in sinusitis. *Journal of Allergy and Clinical Immunology*. 1997;11:489–500.

35. Gibson P, Chang A, Glasgow N, *et al*. Cough in children and adults, diagnosis and assessment: Australian cough guidelines. *Medical Journal of Australia*. 2010;192(5):265–71.

36. Faruqi S, Fahim A, Morice A. Chronic cough and obstructive sleep apnoea: Reflux-associated cough hypersensitivity. *European Respiratory Journal*. 2012;40(4):1049–50.

37. Guimarales K, Drager L, Genta P, *et al*. Effects of oropharyngeal exercises on patients with moderate obstructive sleep apnea syndrome. *American Journal of Respiratory & Critical Care Medicine*. 2009;179:962–6.

38. Gibson PG, Fujimura M, Niimi A. Eosinophilic bronchitis: clinical manifestations and implications for treatment. *Thorax*. 2002;57(2):178–82.

39. Gibson P, Denberg J, Dolovich J, *et al*. Eosinophilic bronchitis without asthma. *The Lancet*. 1989;333(8651):1346–8.

40. Pierce R, Watson T. Psychogenic cough in children: A literature review. *Children's Health Care*. 1998;27(1):63–76.

41. French C, Irwin R, Curley F, Krikorian C. Impact of chronic cough quality of life. *Archives of Internal Medicine*. 1998;158(15):1657–61.

42. Lokshin B, Lindgren S, Weinberger M, Koviach J. Outcome of habit cough in children treated with a brief session of suggestion therapy. *Annals of Allergy*. 1991;67:579–82.

43. McGarvey L, Carton C, Gamble L, *et al*. Prevalence of psychomorbidity among patients with chronic cough. *Cough*. 2006;2(4).

44. Zigmond A, Snaith R. The hospital anxiety and depression scale. *Acta Psychiatrica Scandinavica*. 1983;67(6):361–70.

45. Vertigan A, Theodoros D, Gibson P, Winkworth A. Voice and upper airway symptoms in people with chronic cough and paradoxical vocal fold movement. *Journal of Voice*. 2007;21(3):361–83.

46. Dicipinigaitis P, Tso R, Banauch G. Prevalence of depressive symptoms among patients with chronic cough. *Chest*. 2006;130(6):1839–43.

47. Fulcher R, Cellucci T. Case formulation and behavioural treatment of chronic cough. *Journal of Behavior Therapy and Experimental Psychiatry*. 1997;28(4):291–6.

48. Pinto A, Yanai M, Sekizawa K, *et al.* Conditioned enhancement of cough response in awake guinea pigs. *International Archives of Allergy & Immunology.* 1995;108(1):95–8.

49. Rietveld S, Beest I, Everaerd W. Psychological confounds in medical research: The example of excessive cough in asthma. *Behaviour Research and Therapy.* 2000;38(8):791–800.

50. Brugman S, Newman K. Vocal fold dysfunction. *National Jewish Center for Immunology and Respiratory Medicine.* 1993;11(5):1–5.

51. Mathers-Schmidt B. Paradoxical vocal fold motion: A tutorial on a complex disorder and the speech-language pathologists role. *American Journal of Speech Language Pathology.* 2001;10:111–25.

52. Wamboldt M, Wamboldt F. Psychiatric aspects of respiratory symptoms. In: Taussig L, Landau L (eds). *Pediatric Respiratory Medicine.* St Louis, MO: Mosby; 1999.

53. Ringsberg K, Segesten K, Akerlind I. Walking around in circles ; The life situation of patients with asthma-like symptoms but negative asthma tests. *Scandinavian Journal of Caring Sciences.* 1997;11:103–12.

54. Vertigan AE, Murad MH, Pringsheim T, *et al.* Somatic Cough Syndrome (previously referred to as psychogenic cough) and Tic Cough (previously referred to as habit cough) in adults and children: chest guideline and expert panel report. *Chest.* 2015;9(10):15–0423.

55. Haydour Q, Alahdab F, Farah M, *et al.* Management and diagnosis of psychogenic cough, habit cough, and tic cough: a systematic review. *Chest.* 2014;146(2):355–72.

56. Kardos P. Proposals for a rationale and for rational diagnosis of cough. *Pneumologie.* 2000;54(3):110–5.

57. Irwin R, Glomb W, Chang A. Habit cough, cough tic, and psychogenic cough in adult and paediatric populations: American College of Chest Physicians evidence based clinical practice guidelines. *Chest.* 2006;129(1):174–9.

58. Milgrom H, Corsello P, Freedman M, *et al.* Differential diagnosis and management of chronic cough. *Comprehensive Therapy.* 1990;16(10):46–53.

59. Hutchings H, Eccles R, Smith A, Jawad M. Voluntary cough suppression as an indication of symptom severity in upper respiratory tract infections. *European Respiratory Journal.* 1993;6:1449–54.

60. Farrer J, Keenan J, Levy P. Understanding the pathology and treatment of virus-induced cough. *Home Healthcare Consultant.* 2001;82(2):10–8.

61. McGarvey L, McKeagney P, Polley L, *et al.* Are there clinical features of a sensitized cough reflex? *Pulmonary Pharmacology & Therapeutics.* 2009;22:59–64.

62. Morice A. The cough hypersensitivity syndrome: A novel paradigm for understanding cough. *Lung.* 2010;188(Suppl 1):S87–S90.

63. Morice A, McGarvey L, Dicipinigaitis P. Cough hypersensitivity syndrome is an important clinical concept: A pro/con debate. *Lung.* 2011;190(1):3–9.

64. Pratter M, Brightling C, Boulet L, Irwin R. An empiric integrative approach to the management of cough: ACCP evidence-based clinical practice guidelines. *Chest*. 2006;129(1 Suppl):222S–31S.

65. O'Hara J, Jones N. The aetiology of chronic cough: A review of current theories for the otorhinolaryngologist. *The Journal of Laryngology & Otology*. 2005;119 (7):507.

66. Morice A, Fontana GA, Sovijarvi ARA, *et al*. The diagnosis and management of chronic cough. *European Respiratory Journal*. 2004;24(3):481–92.

67. Lee B, Woo P. Chronic cough as a sign of laryngeal sensory neuropathy: Diagnosis and treatment. *Annals of Otology, Rhinology & Laryngology*. 2005;114(4):253–7.

68. Birring S, Passant C, Patel R, *et al*. Chronic tonsillar enlargement and cough: Preliminary evidence of a novel and treatable cause of chronic cough. *European Respiratory Journal*. 2004;23:199–201.

69. Ryan N, Birring S, Gibson P. Gabapentin for refractory chronic cough: a randomised, double-blind, placebo-controlled trial. *The Lancet*. 2012;380(9853):1583–9.

70. Vertigan AE, Kapela SL, Ryan NM, *et al*. Pregabalin and speech pathology combination therapy for refractory chronic cough: A randomised controlled trial. *Chest*. 2016;149(3): 639–48 .

4

Pulmonary function testing in chronic cough

Peter G. Gibson and Anne E. Vertigan

Most patients with chronic refractory cough will have had pulmonary function testing performed as part of their medical assessment and treatment. Pulmonary function testing is frequently performed in patients with chronic cough and other respiratory disorders. The test measures the ventilatory capacity of the chest and lungs to move gas in and out of the alveoli. It provides an objective assessment of the extent of impairment and is helpful in confirming a diagnosis.[1] Results can indicate whether or not baseline spirometry is normal and whether there is hypersensitivity in the upper or lower airway. Speech pathologists may have variable understanding of pulmonary function testing. The aim of this chapter is to equip the speech pathologist with the tools necessary to interpret pulmonary function test results, and to explain pulmonary function testing and the relevant characteristics in patients with chronic cough. Although interpretation of pulmonary function tests is the role of the respiratory physician, it is useful for the speech pathologist to understand the interpretation of those test results.

Spirometry and pulmonary function testing

Pulmonary function testing typically used in patients with chronic cough involves spirometry, which measures the ventilatory capacity and displacement volume of the lungs. The patient is instructed to take a maximal breath in and then blow into the spirometer for as long and hard as they can. The test is repeated until there are at least two attempts where the Forced Expiratory Volume in one second (FEV_1) results are within 150 ml, and up to eight attempts can be made. Spirometry provides information about both the flow volume loop and absolute values regarding the speed and volume of the movement of air through the airways. The most common indices used are FEV_1, Forced Vital Capacity (FVC), the FEV_1/FVC ratio, and the Peak Expiratory Flow. These indices along with normative values are explained in more detail in Table 4.1. FEV_1 and FEV_1/FVC are measures related to expiratory airflow obstruction, which is typically intrathoracic in origin. FVC provides information on the ability of lung capacity to support respiration and vocalisation.

Measure	Definition	Normative values
FVC	Forced vital capacity. The maximum volume of air that can be exhaled during a forced expiratory manoeuvre.[2]	80–120% of predicted
FEV_1	Forced expired volume in one second. The volume expired in the first second of maximal expiration after a maximal inspiration.[2] Measures the severity of airflow obstruction.	80–120% of predicted
$FEF_{25-75}\%$	The average expired flow over the middle half of the FVC manoeuvre.[2]	80–120% of predicted
FIF_{50}	The flow rate at the 50% point on the total volume inhaled.	
FEV_1/FVC	FEV_1 expressed as a percentage of the FVC and gives a clinically useful index of airflow limitation.	> 70–75%
FEF_{50}/FIF_{50}	The FEF_{50}/FIF_{50} ratio is the ratio of maximal expiratory flow at 50% of the vital capacity and the maximal inspiratory flow at 50% of the vital capacity.	< 1
$PD_{20}FIF_{50}$	Provocation dose of hypertonic saline that causes a 20% reduction in FIF_{50}	
$DRSFIF_{50}$	Dose response slope of inspiratory flow limitation during hypertonic saline provocation.	

Table 4.1: Definitions of commonly used pulmonary function test measures.

The flow volume loop measures flow rate against lung volume, and provides a graphic representation of the patient's spirometry performance during inspiration and expiration.[2] The overall shape of the flow volume loop aids in interpreting the spirometric results.[2] A normal flow volume loop has a rapid initial exhalation phase to peak expiratory flow with a gradual decline in flow back to zero. The inspiratory portion of the loop is a deep curve plotted on the negative portion of the flow axis (Figure 4.1). However, inspiratory data in the flow volume loop is not routinely considered in the interpretation of flow volume loop results.

Spirometric and peak expiratory flow measurements are likely to be normal in patients referred for specialist opinion of chronic cough.[3] The flow volume loop can be used to diagnose asthma as a potential cause of the chronic cough and to identify extrathoracic airway obstruction.[4] In asthma and expiratory airflow obstruction, there is a characteristic concave shape of the expiratory limb of the flow volume loop while the inspiratory limb remains normal (see Figure 4.2).

An obstructive pattern is said to occur when the FEV_1 is low and the FEV_1/FVC ratio is less than 70%. This pattern occurs in asthma, interstitial lung disease and Chronic Obstructive Pulmonary Disease. A restrictive pattern occurs when both FEV_1 and FVC are low. In this situation the FEV_1/FVC ratio may be normal. Restrictive patterns occur in patients with lung scarring. Mixed patterns occur with a very low FEV_1, low FVC and a low FEV_1/FVC ratio. Mixed patterns occur with obesity and musculoskeletal injury.

The flow volume loop is a component of pulmonary function testing and measures the speed and volume of expiration and inspiration. The flow volume loop in individuals with paradoxical vocal fold movement has been shown to have a normal expiratory limb, but attenuation or truncation of the inspiratory limb indicating variable extrathoracic airway obstruction;[5-7] whereas in asthma, the flow volume loop has a normal inspiratory phase, but attenuation in the expiratory phase, indicating variable intrathoracic airflow obstruction. Pulmonary function testing in patients with chronic refractory cough will typically show normal spirometry, with no response to bronchodilators. Provocation testing of the lower airways, known as bronchoprovocation testing, will be negative, however there will be a truncated or flattened inspiratory flow volume loop.[8]

Although spirometry and peak expiratory flow measures are frequently normal in patients with chronic refractory cough, there may be a reduced inspiratory curve which is characteristic of paradoxical vocal fold movement and, in some

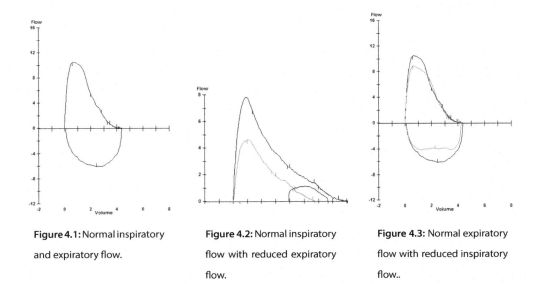

Figure 4.1: Normal inspiratory and expiratory flow.

Figure 4.2: Normal inspiratory flow with reduced expiratory flow.

Figure 4.3: Normal expiratory flow with reduced inspiratory flow..

cases, is a clue that the cough might be due to this condition. Flow volume loops have been used in the assessment and diagnosis of paradoxical vocal fold movement[9] and tend to be normal when patients are asymptomatic.[10] Flow volume loops in paradoxical vocal fold movement have a normal expiratory phase with a plateau configuration in the inspiratory phase,[5] a flattened inspiratory limb,[11] and variable inspiratory flow loops with a characteristic oscillating baseline.[12]

In variable extrathoracic airway obstruction characteristic of paradoxical vocal fold movement, airflow is compromised by dynamic changes in airway calibre. During normal inspiration, airways within the thorax tend to dilate as the lung inflates, while airways outside of the thorax tend to collapse due to the drop in intraluminal pressure. The reverse occurs during expiration, as airways within the thorax collapse but airways outside the thorax are held open by expiratory flow. As a result, variable extrathoracic obstruction primarily affects the inspiratory portion of the flow volume loop. This reduction is shown as a flattening of the usual deep inspiratory curve, while the expiratory portion of the loop appears relatively normal (Figure 4.3 and Figure 4.4).

Airway challenge tests

Airway challenge tests, also known as provocation or hyperresponsiveness tests, are a further development of spirometry. Airway challenge tests are designed to assess the response of the airway to various stimuli. These tests involve pul-

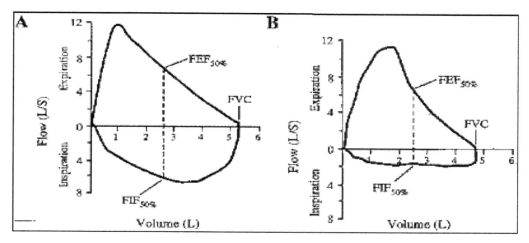

Figure 4.4: Flow volume loop. **A:** Normal inspiratory and expiratory flow. **B:** Normal expiratory flow with truncation of the inspiratory loop.

monary function testing at baseline, followed by administration of a challenge agent and further pulmonary function testing, in order to assess the response to the stimuli. Airway challenge tests can measure both inspiratory and expiratory function and may be direct or indirect.

The flow volume loop assessment can include airway challenge tests involving presentation of noxious substances such as capsaicin, hypertonic saline, histamine or methacholine that act on tissues within the airway in various ways.[13] Several studies have correlated truncation of the inspiratory phase of the flow volume loop and reduced inspiratory flow with glottal constriction.[14–17]

Direct airway challenge tests

Direct airway challenge tests utilise pharmacological agents such as histamine and methacholine that act directly on airway smooth muscle to cause bronchoconstriction.[13] If hyperresponsiveness exists in these smooth muscles, the muscles contract causing airway constriction. Histamine acts on all muscles and structures, whereas methacholine produces bronchoconstriction by stimulating acetylcholine receptors on bronchial smooth muscle cells.[18] These substances provide information about the function of the lower airways but not about the upper airways. They are typically used to diagnose asthma, which is characterised by hyperresponsiveness of the intrathoracic or lower airways.

55

Histamine, manitol, and methacholine are commonly used in cough clinics[3] however, there are several limitations to the use of these substances for provocation testing in chronic refractory cough and paradoxical vocal fold movement. McGarvey[3] claimed that the interpretation of results, particularly when normal, is variable and that results can be affected by the presence of recent upper respiratory tract infection or GERD. Chevalier and Schwartzstein[18] found that over 82% of patients with shortness of breath or cough and a questionable response to inhaled bronchodilators, did not demonstrate airway hyperresponsiveness on the methacholine inhalation challenge. The methacholine inhalation challenge has been reported to result in a false positive for asthma 22% of the time.[19] Chevalier and Schwartzstein[18] suggested that patients with asthma might complain of primary difficulty during inspiration, however did not comment on inspiratory flow during the methacholine inhalation challenge.

Indirect airway challenge tests

Indirect airway challenge tests include the use of hypertonic saline and exercise, which change the osmolarity of airway fluid, trigger mediator release from inflammatory or mast cells and activate airway sensory nerves.[13] The use of hypertonic saline is well standardised in asthma.[20] Studies in healthy individuals with normal lung function have shown a mean percentage fall in FEV_1 plus three standard deviations to be less than 14%.[20] On the basis of this figure a fall in FEV_1 of 15% or more is regarded as abnormal and indicative of asthma. Hypertonic saline has a low false-positive response in healthy individuals.

The use of hypertonic saline to detect extrathoracic or upper airway hyperresponsiveness has been described by several authors,[15–17] where a reduction in inspiratory flow of 20% or more has been correlated with glottal constriction, and is an associated feature in paradoxical vocal fold movement. The hypertonic saline challenge can be used to trigger upper airway closure. An abnormal result will be a fall in FIF_{50} of greater than 20%.

An advantage of provocation testing is that standardised provocation testing protocols can be employed,[15] thus ensuring consistency amongst large participant groups. Figure 4.4 provides an example of this phenomenon, with Figure 4.4A depicting a normal hypertonic saline challenge result and Figure 4.4B depicting a plateau configuration of the inspiratory limb of the flow volume loop following provocation with hypertonic saline.

Abnormal hypertonic saline challenge results are present in a high proportion of patients with laryngeal dysfunction syndromes. We compared hypertonic saline challenge results between patients with a range of laryngeal conditions. Abnormal results were present in 57% with refractory chronic cough, 80% with paradoxical vocal fold movement, 25% with globus pharyngeus, and 40% with muscle tension dysphonia.[21]

Exercise can also provoke an upper and lower airway response,[22] however the stimulus is difficult to quantify. Some researchers use a percentage of maximum heart rate as a target during exercise challenge. Thus, airway provocation with hypertonic saline may be a useful test to study both upper and lower airway responsiveness given the effect on mast cell and sensory nerve activation. Some authors reported using airway challenge tests to rule out hyperresponsiveness of the lower airway in order to differentially diagnose paradoxical vocal fold movement from asthma.[10]

Informal inhalation or exercise challenges can also be performed. These challenges involve baseline spirometry, followed by exposure to the challenge stimulus, and then repeat spirometry. Examples of challenge stimuli include chlorox, ammonia, running up stairs and perfumes. The advantage of this informal procedure is that it is often easy to administer; however, it is difficult to quantify the stimulus dose.

Cough reflex sensitivity testing

Cough reflex sensitivity testing is an objective test. It involves administration of known tussive substances such as capsaicin, citric acid or tartaric acid, and measuring the cough response. In capsaicin testing, a standard dose of capsaicin is administered via a nebuliser and the cough response for the following 30 seconds is measured. The dose ranges from 0.87 to 500 u/mol. These doses are administered until the individual coughs five times. Three measurements are taken during this test including:

1. Cough Threshold: The lowest dose of capsaicin required to elicit a single cough.
2. C2: The dose of capsaicin required to elicit two coughs.
3. C5: The dose of capsaicin required to elicit five coughs. A normal result is 500 u/mol.

During this test, an urge to cough may be experienced at a dose lower than that required to elicit a cough.

In addition to providing objective measurements regarding the sensitivity of the cough reflex, this test provides opportunities for the speech pathologist to observe the patient's cough behaviour in the presence of a known tussive stimulus. The patient's cough response to the stimulus, along with their attempts to suppress cough, provide valuable insights for behavioural management of cough.

The instructions used during the capsaicin cough challenge can help to differentiate between the thresholds for voluntary and reflexive cough. If the patient is instructed to try to suppress their cough as much as possible, the dose at which a cough is elicited is rated as the reflexive cough threshold. In contrast, if the patient is instructed to cough when they need to, the dose at which a cough is elicited is thought to be the voluntary cough threshold.

Oximetry

Oxygen saturation levels are frequently measured in patients presenting with respiratory distress, particularly in the emergency department. Oximetry remains normal during acute episodes of paradoxical vocal fold movement.[23] Normal oximetry indicates that the individual is inspiring sufficient air. In contrast, oxygen saturation levels are usually reduced in patients experiencing respiratory distress due to a lower airway restriction or obstruction.

Induced sputum

Induced sputum is a test used to detect eosinophilic bronchitis.[24,25] This procedure is rarely available outside specialist clinics. Induced sputum is not a routine investigation for chronic refractory cough and empiric trials of corticosteroids are often substituted for the procedure.

Summary

Pulmonary function testing is commonly used by respiratory physicians to assess respiratory function. Familiarity with pulmonary function testing results provides the speech pathologist with more thorough knowledge of respiratory function when working with this population. The addition of provocation testing with pulmonary function testing is valuable in the diagnosis of paradoxical vocal fold movement and laryngeal hyperresponsiveness.

References

1. Johns T, Crocket A. Lung function testing. In: Gibson P (ed). *Evidence Based Respiratory Medicine*: BMJ Publishing Group; 2004.

2. Pierce R, Johns D. Spirometry: The measurement and interpretation of ventilatory function in clinical practice: *Thoracic Society of Australia and New Zealand*; 1995.

3. McGarvey L. Cough 6: Which investigations are most useful in the diagnosis of chronic cough? *Thorax*. 2004;59:342–6.

4. Irwin R, Pratter M, Holland R, *et al*. Postnasal drip causes cough and is associated with reversible upper airway obstruction. *Chest*. 1984;85(3):346–52.

5. Nagai A, Yamaguchi E, Sakamoto K, Takahashi E. Functional upper airway obstruction. *Chest*. 1992;101:1460–1.

6. Wamboldt M, Wamboldt F. Psychiatric aspects of respiratory symptoms. In: Taussig L, Landau L (eds). *Pediatric Respiratory Medicine*. St Louis, MO: Mosby; 1999.

7. Bahrainwala A, Simon M. Wheezing and vocal cord dysfunction mimicking asthma. *Current Opinion in Pulmonary Medicine*. 2001;7(1):8–13.

8. Morris M, Christopher K. Diagnostic criteria for the classification of vocal cord dysfunction. *Chest*. 2010;138(5):1213–23.

9. Lacy T, McManis S. Psychogenic stridor. *General Hospital Psychiatry*. 1994;16:213–23.

10. Mathers-Schmidt B. Paradoxical vocal fold motion: A tutorial on a complex disorder and the speech-language pathologist's role. *American Journal of Speech Language Pathology*. 2001;10:111–25.

11. Maschka D, Hoffman H. Paradoxical vocal fold dysfunction and laryngeal asthma. *Current Opinion in Otolaryngology & Head and Neck Surgery*. 1999;7(6):339.

12. Marsh C, Trudeau M, Weiland J. Recurrent asthma despite corticosteroid therapy in a 35 year old woman. *Chest*. 1994;105:1855–7.

13. deMeer G. Airway responsiveness to direct and indirect stimuli: A population based approach. Doctoral Thesis, Universiteit Utrecht, The Netherlands; 1961.

14. Bucca C, Rolla G, Scappaticci E, *et al*. Extrathoracic and intrathoracic airway responsiveness in sinusitis. *Journal of Allergy and Clinical Immunology*. 1995;95(1):52–7.

15. Gibson P, Taramarcaz P, Borgas T. Evaluation of diagnostic tests for vocal cord dysfunction. *American Journal of Respiratory and Critical Care Medicine*. 2004;169:A317.

16. Taramarcaz P, Grissell T, Borgas T, Gibson P. Transient post-viral vocal cord dysfunction. *Journal of Allergy and Clinical Immunology*. 2004;114(6):1471–2.

17. Ryan N, Gibson P. Cough reflex hypersensitivity and upper airway hyperresponsiveness in vocal cord dysfunction with chronic cough. *Respirology*. 2006;11 (Suppl 2):A48.

18. Chevalier B, Schwartzstein R. Methacholine challenge testing: Defining its diagnostic role. *The Journal of Respiratory Diseases*. 2001;22(3):153–62.

19. Irwin R, Curley F, French C. Chronic cough: The spectrum and frequency of causes, key components of the diagnostic evaluation and outcome of specific thearpy. *American Review of Respiratory Disease*. 1990;141:640–7.

20. Anderson S, Gibson P. Use of aerosols of hypertonic saline and distilled water (Fog). In: Barnes P, Grunstein M, Leff A, Woolcock A (eds). *Asthma* (volume 4). Philadephia, PA: Lippincott Raven Publishers; 1997.

21. Vertigan A, Bone S, Gibson PG. Laryngeal sensory dysfunction in Laryngeal Hypersensitivity Syndrome. *Respirology*. 2013;18(6):948–56.

22. Morris M, Deal L, Bean D, *et al*. Vocal cord dysfunction in patients with exertional dyspnoea. *Chest*. 1999;116:1676–82.

23. Balkissoon R, Kenn K. Asthma: Vocal cord dysfunction (VCD) and other dysfunctional breathing disorders. *Seminars in Respiratory and Critical Care Medicine*. 2012;33(6):595–605.

24. Gibson P, Denberg J, Dolovich J, *et al*. Eosinophilic bronchitis without asthma. *The Lancet*. 1989;333(8651):1346–8.

25. McGarvey L. Cough 6: Which invetigations are most useful in the diagnois of chronic cough? *Thorax*. 2004;59:342–6.

5

Otolaryngology management of chronic cough

Kenneth W. Altman

Background

Chronic cough is a challenging clinical problem to manage for a number of reasons, including: (1) the list of possible contributing factors makes a specific causative diagnosis difficult, (2) multifactorial etiologies may lead to synergistic effects exacerbating the cough, (3) patients often have a prolonged course with inconsistent treatments using 'polypharmacy', and (4) many care providers may be involved, yet there may not be a defined leader of the care team. While the behavior of coughing and maladaptive mechanisms (such as laryngospasm and paradoxical vocal fold motion) may be managed by the speech pathologist, it is also important to fully assess and manage medical contributions to the cough.

There is a significant epidemiologic impact of chronic cough, with a prevalence estimated by surveys to be 9–33% of the population. In 2006, US$3.6 billion was spent on over the counter cough and cold medications. In the 2010 United States National Ambulatory Medical Care Survey (NAMCS), there were 30 million outpatient visits for acute and chronic cough, accounting for about 3% of visits to all physicians. For patients, chronic cough can lead to significantly decreased quality of life from a physical and psychological standpoint.[1]

Otolaryngologists have a special interest in patients with cough, as we routinely care for many of the associated conditions. Cough is categorized as acute (lasting < 3 weeks), subacute (3–8 weeks), and chronic (> 8 weeks). Acute cough is most commonly due to viral upper respiratory tract infection (URTI), asthma or pulmonary exacerbation, acute exposure to an environmental irritant, or an acute cardiopulmonary condition such as bronchitis and pneumonia. Subacute cough is most commonly due to lingering effects following an acute URTI, but may also include *Bordetella pertussis* and *Mycoplasma* infections. Chronic cough is the more commonly seen by the otolaryngologist, whose contributions can be multifactorial and synergistic.[10] For example, up to 93% of troublesome coughs have been shown to have more than one etiology.[11]

The primary diseases associated with chronic cough and managed by otolaryngologists are rhinologic and esophageal-related. Here, the cough reflex is considered protective especially when the normal mucocilliary transport mechanism is inadequate or overwhelmed.[2] The reflex is a coordinated release of air with intrathoracic pressures as high as 300 mm Hg and air velocities up to 500 miles per hour. Figure 5.1 outlines the major contributions to chronic cough, with the act of coughing centered in the larynx.

Rhinologic contributions may be allergic or non-allergic irritant exposures to the nasal passages which produce inflammation, outflow tract obstruction and production of inflamed mucus. This also leads to mucus stasis, bacterial overgrowth and the pathogenesis of sinusitis. The concept of the *unified airway* is an integral component to understanding and treating cough.[3] The unified airway refers to the close relationship of the upper and lower airways, with multiple physical and physiologic links. For example, allergy triggers both upper and lower airway disease and exacerbates asthma. Also, sinus disease can have the same result in addition to seeding infection to the lungs to induce bronchitis.[4] Although pulmonary disease is beyond the scope of this chapter, the *unified airway* concept emphasizes the importance of interdisciplinary care of the patient.

Gastroesophageal reflux disease (GERD) and laryngopharyngeal reflux (LPR) are similarly important to the otolaryngologist. These diseases may present with the overlapping symptoms of chronic non-productive cough, throat-clearing behavior, and globus sensation, but may also lead to increased laryngeal hypersensitivity and have been associated with 'the irritable larynx', laryngospasm, and paradoxical vocal fold motion (PVFM). Here, GERD/LPR can induce cough by directly irritating the sensory receptors in the larynx at the time of regurgitation, but can also leave a residue of pepsin on the laryngeal mucosa to cause ongoing auto-digestion and increased sensitivity to other episodes of reflux. The tissue effects at the level of the larynx include direct inflammation, passing of materials through this region, or development of secondary

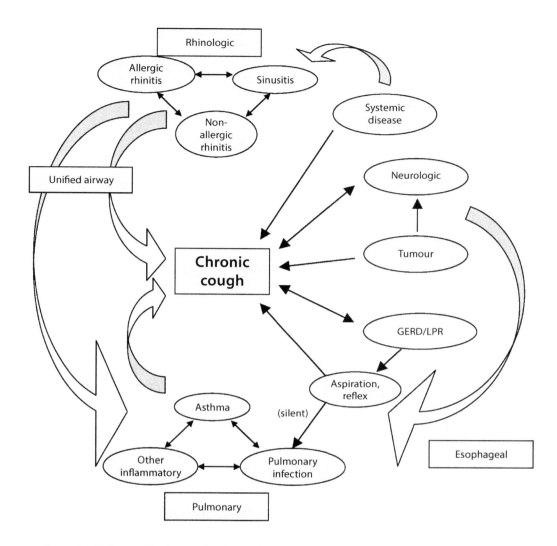

Figure 5.1: Major contributions to chronic cough.

edema.[3] Gross or micro-aspiration may also ensue from reflux that can induce a pneumonitis, triggering a pulmonary-based cough. Also, the act of coughing itself can induce regurgitation and reflux through the connection of the lower esophageal sphincter at the diaphragm.

Examples of systemic disease resulting in cough include most commonly the use of angiotensin converting enzyme inhibitors (ACEi) for hypertension where the ACEi can result in cough in as many as 3–10% of patients. Congestive heart failure should also be considered through pulmonary congestion. Autoimmune diseases including sarcoidosis and granulomatosis with polyangitis (formerly

Wegener's granulomatosis) can manifest with both nasal and pulmonary disease. Other autoimmune disease such as dermatomyositis and scleroderma result in esophageal dysmotility and increased association with GERD and LPR. The use of oral corticosteroids for these disorders also predisposes to susceptibility to infections, among other consequences.

The initial evaluation

Cough is a nonspecific symptom with a large differential diagnosis, so an organized approach focusing first on the duration is essential to effective management.[6,7] Also, a productive (versus dry cough) is more likely associated with an infectious or allergic etiology, rather than reflux-related or neurogenic.[8] Cough may be related to living or working environments, such as allergies, irritants, chemicals, dust, and exposure to tobacco smoke (a significant trigger for chronic cough). A review of medications should always be performed to determine use of ACEi.

Questioning the patient should include typical or atypical symptoms related to the most common causes of chronic cough: rhinosinus disease, GERD/LPR, asthma, and non-eosinophillic bronchitis.[9] Particular attention should be paid to any 'alarm' symptoms, things that may point to a serious life threatening condition. Alarm symptoms include syncope, rib fracture, pneumonia, hemoptysis, stridor, and palpitations, among others. Patients with these symptoms may need acute care and should bypass the routine cough management paradigm.

The physical exam for patients with chronic cough includes a full head and neck exam, auscultation of the lungs, and nasopharyngeal laryngoscopy. Ears should be examined for manifestations of allergies including retracted tympanic membranes or serous otitis media. The neck should be examined for lymphadenopathy that may suggest infection or malignancy. On nasopharyngeal laryngoscopy, some findings may be readily apparent, such as, signs of infection, tumors, or motility issues. Often, however, findings just reveal a trail of inflammation or irritation. Special attention should be paid to the color, vascularity, and presence of edema on the mucosal lining from the nasal cavity to the larynx. Chronic inflammation can lead to lymphoid hyperplasia and 'cobblestoning', or significant mucus secretion.[12]

The laryngeal examination should be performed systematically. Again, mucus secretions, mucosal lining, and patterns of erythema and edema should be noted. Evidence of pooled secretions or laryngeal penetration may be warning signs for aspiration. The laryngeal anatomy can be broken into subsites to help objectively document findings. A complete laryngeal examination should include active phonation and quiet breathing. Mobility, symmetry, and closure of the true vocal folds should be assessed. The subglottis may be inspected in a cooperative patient with proper positioning and local anesthesia. Although this is not a routine manner to evaluate the subglottis, it can provide a glimpse at the laryngeal subsite.

Establishing a differential diagnosis

Following a targeted history and physical examination including endoscopy, it is ideal to structure a differential diagnosis prior to starting empiric therapy or determining the need for further objective testing.

Acute cough < 3 weeks

The most common cause of the acute cough is an upper respiratory tract infection (URTI). Influenza, parainfluenza, adenovirus, rhinovirus, and respiratory syncytial virus are among the most common viral pathogens. Cough associated with a URTI's is most prevalent (83%) in the first 48 hours and diminishes to 26% over the course of the next two weeks.[22] Even chest x-ray for acute URTI has a low yield with normal findings in 97%.[23] URTI associated cough can be managed symptomaticaly, despite little evidence of specific pharmacologic effect.[7] Antitussive agents may also be effective.[7,24,25] Exacerbations of chronic diseases such as asthma, chronic obstructive pulmonary disease, allergies, and the initial catarrhal stages of *Bordetella pertussis* can also cause an acute cough. Although rarely an isolated symptom, acute cough can present in patients with pneumonia, congestive heart failure, and even pulmonary embolism.

Subacute cough 3–8 weeks

The first objective is to determine if the cough is post-infectious, since non-infectious etiologies are likely to be multifactorial and can have similar causes of chronic cough.[2] Post-infectious cough is thought to be from extensive disruption of epithelial integrity and widespread airway inflammation of the upper and/or lower airways with or without transient hyperresponsiveness.[26] Increased secretions produced secondary to the level of inflammation continue to stimulate the cough reflex.[22] Gastroesophageal reflux may also play a role in subacute cough. Repeated forceful cough causes increases in abdominal pressure that may aggravate preexisting reflux disease.[26]

Bordetella pertussis or 'whooping cough' is a highly contagious, unique cause of post-infectious cough with characteristic biphasic cough, 'whoop', or cough-vomit syndrome.[26] Despite childhood immunization, there appears to have been a recent resurgence, even in adult patients.[27] Erythromycin or trimethoprim/sulfamethoxazole are the treatments of choice, but if initiated during the paroxysmal stage have limited benefit.[28] Symptomatic control of the paroxysmal cough with beta-agonist, corticosteroids, and antihistamines has been shown to have no benefit and is not recommended.[26]

Chronic cough > 8 weeks

Angiotensin-Converting Enzyme (ACE) inhibitors

In 2010, ACE inhibitors were the fifth most commonly prescribed drug class in the United States, accounting for 168 million prescriptions.[14] The incidence of cough has been reported anywhere from 0.2% to 33%,[10] and the cough is usually described as 'dry' or 'tickly' and is not dose dependent.[15] The cough can begin at anywhere between the first dose and years after initiation of treatment. Once discontinued, the median time for resolution of the cough has been shown to be 26 days.[15] It is important to partner with the patient's other physicians to ensure proper alternative treatment of their medical conditions.

Irritant induced cough

An irritant is a chemical that is not corrosive, but causes a reversible inflammatory effect on tissue at this site of contact.[16] Irritants are among the most common causes of cough in patients with normal chest radiographs.[17] Cigarette smoking is the most common irritant, which results in ciliary dysfunction, mucus stasis, and cough receptor stimulation. Effects are dose dependent, and prevalence of cough returns to near normal in ex-smokers.[18–20] Workers with occupational exposure to low molecular weight particles have also been shown to have an increased incidence of cough.[13] The collapse of the World Trade Center towers following the terrorist attacks in 2001 caused exposure to inorganic dust, polyaromatic hydrocarbons, and a complex mixture of other irritants, resulting in persisting cough and nonspecific airway hyperreactivity.[21] Removal of the irritant should be the initial step in management in these patients.

Upper Airway Cough Syndrome (UACS)

UACS alone, or in conjunction with other conditions has been found to be the most common cause of chronic cough, and includes the generic consortium of issues contributing to 'post nasal drip'.[31] Sinonasal conditions may be irritant, infectious, or allergic in etiology and represent a true reflection of the unified airway model.[3] On exam, the nasopharynx or oropharynx may show mucoid or mucopurulent secretions with 'cobblestoning' of the mucosa to indicate chronic inflammation.[32] Not all patients feel postnasal drip, and the described clinical picture is neither sensitive nor specific.[2] When a component of allergic rhinitis exists, avoidance of the allergen is ideal, along with nasal steroids, antihistamines, and/or cromolyn as initial drugs of choice.[33] Immunotherapy for desensitization is also an option, but does not give immediate relief. For infectious sinusitis, intranasal steroid should be combined with an antibiotic and a short-term nasal decongestant may be used.

Gastroesophageal Reflux Disease (GERD)

Understanding the relationship between GERD and laryngopharyngeal reflux (LPR) with cough is still evolving, however both involve retrograde flow of gastric contents past the lower esophageal sphincter (LES).[34,35] Refluxed contents are not limited to acid and may include bile and pepsin, which are also implicated in laryngeal irritation.[36,37] An esophageal-bronchial reflex in the mucosa of the distal esophagus can also stimulate chronic cough.[38] The prevalence of GERD related chronic cough has increased from 10% in 1981, to 36% in 1998,[39] and is one of the most common causes of chronic cough. While patients with daily heartburn and regurgitation[38] should be suspected of having reflux, these symptoms are only present in about half of patients with reflux. Reflux should be suspected in patients that have cough in the morning, after eating, and with phonation. Medications, food and lifestyle are all potential contributing factors to reflux, and should be recognized as components of the treatment plan.[39] Findings of erythema and edema of the true folds, interarytenoid mucosa, arytenoids, and posterior pharyngeal wall have been shown to be associated with reflux, however these findings may also be due to trauma from cough itself.[40,41]

Treatment with a proton pump inhibitor (PPI) is currently the mainstay of initial management, along with aliginates which form a gelatinous barrier on the gastric contents which reduces regurgitation. Prokinetic medication such as metoclopramide and domperidone (not sold in the US) have been shown to control cough and hoarseness when combined with PPI in the majority of patients, but it has limited use due to the side effect profile.[35]

Pulmonary etiologies

The spectrum of pulmonary disease related to chronic cough is reviewed elsewhere, but still bears mention. Asthma accounts for 24% to 29% of chronic cough in non-smoking adults,[10] and may be the only presenting symptom in patients with cough variant asthma (CVA).[45] The cough reflex in CVA patients is stronger than in patients with typical asthma, and hyperresponsiveness to methacholine is less. Nonasthmatic eosinophilic bronchitis (NAEB) is defined as cough with no airflow obstruction, normal airway hyperresponsiveness, and sputum eosinophilia (> 3% nonsquamous sputum eosinophils).[46] The etiology of asthma and NAEB is unknown but can be associated with exposure to inhaled aeroallergen or an occupational sensitizer.[47]

It is recommended by the American College of Chest Physicians (ACCP) that patients with suspected asthma but normal pulmonary function testing undergo methacholine inhalation challenge (MIC), which can rule out asthma as the etiology of cough (high negative predictive value).[48–53]

Syndromes associated with chronic productive cough include chronic bronchitis, bronchiectasis, and bronchiolitis. Chronic bronchitis is a disease characterized by an abnormal inflammatory response to gases and particles such as cigarette smoking. When there is airflow obstruction seen on spirometry, it is termed chronic obstructive pulmonary disease (COPD). In bronchiectasis, mucopurulent sputum is seen from chronic inflammation and infection due to chronic bronchial wall damage. A spectrum of processes can be at play in bronchiolitis, with small airways affected by infectious, postinfectious, inflammatory, or idiopathic processes. These etiologies should be managed in partnership with a pulmonologist for accuracy of diagnosis.

Management and the complicated diagnosis

The chronic cough patient who does not respond to the initial line of empiric therapy can be very challenging. Many of them have seen multiple physicians without significant relief, and up to 23% of those referred to a cough specialist have been misdiagnosed with psychogenic cough.[10] The initial step in the management process for chronic cough should be to eliminate ACEi and obtain chest radiography, noting any findings as a potential cause of the cough, and

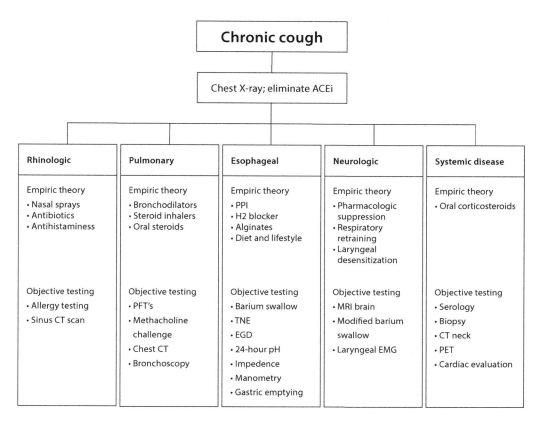

Figure 5.2: An algorithmic approach to diagnosis.[30]

pulmonologist consultation should be considered.[6] Based on the complexity of care, a systematic approach with objective testing should be considered, remembering that over two-thirds of chronic cough patients have multifactorial etiologies.

Figure 5.2 demonstrates an algorithmic approach, adapted from formal recommendations of the American College of Chest Physicians.[30] Following initial evaluation and failure of empiric therapy, objective testing should proceed for etiologies contributing to the cough with prioritizing those areas of major clinical suspicion. Rhinologic causes related to allergic or infectious disease can be readily identified through formal allergy testing or sinus CT scan. Failure of response to aggressive medical therapy may warrant allergy immunotherapy/densensitization, or endoscopic sinus surgery.

Objective testing for pulmonary etiologies may include formal pulmonary function testing (PFT), methacholine challenge, chest CT, and formal bronchoscopy with cell washings. Bronchoscopy is especially important when obtaining definitive diagnosis for endobronchial mass lesions and NAEB.[46]

Chronic cough presumed related to reflux disease that is refractory to empiric management requires objective testing. Barium esophagram evaluates for dysmotility, strictures, and some esophageal lining disease but it's sensitivity for reflux is as low as 33% in some studies.[42] Esophagoscopy allows for examination of the esophageal lining and aids in the diagnosis of esophagitis, Barrett's esophagus, and esophageal malignancy, although it is paramount to recognize that absence of esophagitis does not rule out reflux as the cause of the cough.

Twenty-four hour pH probe testing with impedance (or 48-hour Bravo capsule placement in the mid-esophagus) determines the presence of pathologic regurgitation and can be associated with the timing of coughing. Impedance testing distinguishes between acid and non-acid reflux, where the latter causes longer lasting symptoms.[43,44] There also needs to be a stated goal of the test. For example, these tests should be done off reflux pharmacotherapy if the goals are to determine proof that reflux is contributing to the cough, determine baseline severity of disease, and determine candidacy for laparoscopic Nissen fundoplication. However, testing on reflux medication may be of use to determine adequacy of pharmacotherapy to control the disease. Surgical management for reflux should also be considered in select patients.[39]

There is a fairly broad array of neurologic and systemic diseases that can cause cough, and the concept of 'neurogenic cough' due to post-viral syndromes is a diagnosis of exclusion. In cases of paradoxical vocal fold motion and laryngospasm associated with chronic cough, a speech language pathologist can assess behavioral manifestations of symptoms and treat with breath control techniques.[29] Roles also exist for pharmacologic cough suppression, laryngeal electromyography (EMG) in cases of vocal paresis, and modified Barium swallow when aspiration is suspected. Evaluation of systemic disease as it may contribute to chronic cough often involves extensive serology, but may also include cardiac evaluation, and Positron Emission Tomography (PET) in the case of malignancy. The complicated chronic cough patient therefore requires interdisciplinary care, exclusion of occult malignancy, and often ongoing management.

Summary

There are numerous potential sources of chronic cough, which is often multifactorial, so a systematic approach is advised. The first objective should be to filter out obvious diagnoses such as cancer, aspiration, neurogenic, and systemic diseases with a good history and physical. Next, elimination of obvious sources such as ACEi use or smoking should be recommended. Stratification of cough, based on duration, will then allow for a more manageable differential diagnosis. If empiric treatment fails to resolve the cough, then objective testing is warranted. Patient care is optimized with a collaborative effort from a multidisciplinary team using a systematic approach.

References

1.   Altman KW, Irwin RS. Cough: a new frontier in otolaryngology. *Otolaryngology - Head and Neck Surgery*. 2011;144(3):348–52.

2.   Madison JM, Irwin RS. Cough: a worldwide problem. *Otolaryngologic Clinics of North America*. 2010;43(1):1–13, vii.

3.   Krouse JH, Altman KW. Rhinogenic laryngitis, cough, and the unified airway. *Otolaryngologic Clinics of North America*. 2010;43(1):111–21.

4.   Krouse JH. The unified airway–conceptual framework. *Otolaryngologic Clinics of North America*. 2008;41(2):257–66, v.

5.   Kuzniar TJ, Morgenthaler TI, Afessa B, Lim KG. Chronic cough from the patient's perspective. *Mayo Clinic Proceedings*. 2007;82(1):56–60.

6.   Irwin RS, Baumann MH, Bolser DC, *et al*. Diagnosis and management of cough executive summary: ACCP evidence-based clinical practice guidelines. *Chest*. 2006;129(1 Suppl):1S–23S.

7.   Morice AH, McGarvey L, Pavord I, British Thoracic Society Cough Guideline Group. Recommendations for the management of cough in adults. *Thorax*. 2006;61 Suppl 1:i1–24.

8.   Cerveri I, Accordini S, Corsico A, *et al*. Chronic cough and phlegm in young adults. 1European Respiratory Journal. 2003;22(3):413–7.

9.   Irwin RS, Madison JM. The persistently troublesome cough. *American Journal of Respiratory and Critical Care Medicine*. 2002;165(11):1469–74.

10. Irwin RS, Curley FJ, French CL. Chronic cough. The spectrum and frequency of causes, key components of the diagnostic evaluation, and outcome of specific therapy. *The American Review of Respiratory Disease*. 1990;141(3):640–7.

11. Irwin RS, Boulet LP, Cloutier MM, *et al*. Managing cough as a defense mechanism and as a symptom. A consensus panel report of the American College of Chest Physicians. *Chest*.1998 114:133S–81S.

12. Rubin BK. Mucus and mucins. *Otolaryngologic Clinics of North America*. 2010;43(1):27–34, vii–viii.

13. Morice AH. Epidemiology of cough. Pulmonary *Pharmacology & Therapeutics*. 2002;15(3):253–9.

14. 2010_Top_Therapeutic_Classes_by_RX.pdf. imshealth.com. Available at: http://www.imshealth.com/deployedfiles/ims/Global/Content/Corporate/Press%20Room/Top-line%20Market%20

Data/2010%20Top-line%20Market%20Data/2010_Top_Therapeutic_Classes_by_RX.pdf. [Accessed January 4, 2012].

15. Lacourcière Y, Brunner H, Irwin R, *et al*. Effects of modulators of the renin-angiotensin-aldosterone system on cough. Losartan Cough Study Group. *Journal of Hypertension*. 1994;12(12):1387–93.

16. US Department of Labor. The OSHA Hazard Communication Standard (HCS) Regulations (Standards-29 CFR). USA, Occupational Safety and Health Administration (OSHA). Appendix A to the Hazard Communication Standard, 1994.

17. Pavord ID, Wardlaw AJ. The A to E of airway disease. *Clinical & Experimental Allergy*. 2010;40(1):62–7.

18. Jansen DF, Schouten JP, Vonk JM, *et al*. Smoking and airway hyperresponsiveness especially in the presence of blood eosinophilia increase the risk to develop respiratory symptoms: a 25-year follow-up study in the general adult population. *American Journal of Respiratory and Critical Care Medicine*. 1999;160(1):259–64.

19. Janson C, Chinn S, Jarvis D, *et al*. Effect of passive smoking on respiratory symptoms, bronchial responsiveness, lung function, and total serum IgE in the European Community Respiratory Health Survey: a cross-sectional study. *Lancet*. 2001;358(9299):2103–9.

20. Larsson ML, Loit HM, Meren M, *et al*. Passive smoking and respiratory symptoms in the FinEsS Study. *European Respiratory Journal*. 2003;21(4):672–6.

21. Brooks SM. Occupational, environment, and irritant-induced cough. *Otolaryngological Clinics of North America*. 2010; (43):85–96.

22. Curley FJ, Irwin RS, Pratter MR, *et al*. Cough and the common cold. *American Review of Respiratory Disease*. 1988;138(2):305–11.

23. Diehr P, Wood RW, Bushyhead J, *et al*. Prediction of pneumonia in outpatients with acute cough–a statistical approach. *Journal of Chronic Diseases*. 1984;37(3):215–25.

24. Bolser DC. Pharmacologic management of cough. *Otolaryngologic Clinics of North America*. 2010;43(1):147–55, xi.

25. Pavord ID, Chung KF. Management of chronic cough. *Lancet*. 2008;371(9621):1375–84.

26. Braman SS. Postinfectious cough: ACCP evidence-based clinical practice guidelines. *Chest*. 2006;129(1 Suppl):138S–46S.

27. Rohani P, Drake JM. The decline and resurgence of pertussis in the US. *Epidemics*. 2011;3(3–4):183–188.

28. Hoppe JE. Comparison of erythromycin estolate and erythromycin ethylsuccinate for treatment of pertussis. The Erythromycin Study Group. *The Pediatric Infectious Disease Journal*. 1992;11(3):189–93.

29. Murry T and Sapienza C. The role of voice therapy in the management of paradoxical vocal fold motion, chronic cough, and laryngospasm. *Otolaryngologic Clinics of North America*. 2010;43(1):43–66.

30. Irwin RS. Unexplained cough in the adult. *Otolaryngologic Clinics of North America*. 2010;43(1):167–80, xi–xii.

31. Smyrnios NA, Irwin RS, Curley FJ, French CL. From a prospective study of chronic cough: diagnostic and therapeutic aspects in older adults. *Archives of Internal Medicine*. 1998;158(11):1222.

32. Pratter MR. Chronic upper airway cough syndrome secondary to rhinosinus diseases (previously referred to as postnasal drip syndrome): ACCP evidence-based clinical practice guidelines. *Chest*. 2006;129(1 Suppl):63S–71S.

33. Naclerio RM. Allergic rhinitis. *New England Journal of Medicine*. 1991;325(12):860–9.

34. Koufman JA. Laryngopharyngeal reflux is different from classic gastroesophageal reflux disease. *Ear Nose Throat Journal*. 2002;81(9 Suppl 2):7–9.

35. Merati AL. Reflux and cough. Otolaryngologic Clinics of North America. 2010;43(1):97–110, ix.

36. Adhami T, Goldblum JR, Richter JE, Vaezi MF. The role of gastric and duodenal agents in laryngeal injury: an experimental canine model. *American Journal of Gastroenterology*. 2004;99(11):2098–106.

37. Johnston N, Dettmar PW, Bishwokarma B, *et al*. Activity/stability of human pepsin: implications for reflux attributed laryngeal disease. *The Laryngoscope*. 2007;117(6):1036–9.

38. Irwin RS, French CL, Curley FJ, *et al*. Chronic cough due to gastroesophageal reflux. Clinical, diagnostic, and pathogenetic aspects. *Chest*. 1993;104(5):1511–7.

39. Irwin RS. Chronic cough due to gastroesophageal reflux disease: ACCP evidence-based clinical practice guidelines. *Chest*. 2006;129(1 Suppl):80S–94S.

40. Hanson DG, Jiang J, Chi W. Quantitative color analysis of laryngeal erythema in chronic posterior laryngitis. *Journal of Voice*. 1998;12(1):78–83.

41. Park W, Hicks DM, Khandwala F, *et al*. Laryngopharyngeal reflux: prospective cohort study evaluating optimal dose of proton-pump inhibitor therapy and pretherapy predictors of response. *The Laryngoscope*. 2005;115(7):1230–8.

42. Richter JE, Castell DO. Gastroesophageal reflux. Pathogenesis, diagnosis, and therapy. *Annals of Internal Medicine*. 1982;97(1):93–103.

43. Sifrim D, Dupont L, Blondeau K, *et al*. Weakly acidic reflux in patients with chronic unexplained cough during 24 hour pressure, pH, and impedance monitoring. *Gut*. 2005;54(4):449–454.

44. Agrawal A, Roberts J, Sharma N, *et al*. Symptoms with acid and nonacid reflux may be produced by different mechanisms. *Diseases of the Esophagus*. 2009;22(5):467–70.

45. Corrao WM, Braman SS, Irwin RS. Chronic cough as the sole presenting manifestation of bronchial asthma. *New England Journal of Medicine*. 1979;300(12):633–7.

46. Brightling CE, Ward R, Goh KL, *et al*. Eosinophilic bronchitis is an important cause of chronic cough. *American Journal of Respiratory and Critical Care Medicine*. 1999;160(2):406–10.

47. Berry MA, Hargadon B, McKenna S, *et al*. Observational study of the natural history of eosinophilic bronchitis. *Clinical and Experimental Allergy*. 2005;35(5):598–601.

48. Crapo RO, Casaburi R, Coates AL, *et al*. Guidelines for methacholine and exercise challenge testing-1999. This official statement of the American Thoracic Society was adopted by the ATS Board of Directors, July 1999. *American Journal of Respiratory and Critical Care Medicine*. 2000;161(1):309–29.

49. Dicpinigaitis PV. Chronic cough due to asthma: ACCP evidence-based clinical practice guidelines. *Chest*. 2006;129(1_suppl):75S–79S.

50. Cheriyan S, Greenberger PA, Patterson R. Outcome of cough variant asthma treated with inhaled steroids. *Annals of Allergy, Asthma and Immunology*. 1994;73(6):478–80.

51. Irwin RS, French CT, Smyrnios NA, Curley FJ. Interpretation of positive results of a methacholine inhalation challenge and 1 week of inhaled bronchodilator use in diagnosing and treating cough-variant asthma. *Archives of Internal Medicine*. 1997;157(17):1981–7.

52. Brightling CE. Chronic cough due to nonasthmatic eosinophilic bronchitis: ACCP evidence-based clinical practice guidelines. *Chest*. 2006;129(1 Suppl):116S–121S.

53. Braman SS and Abu-Hijileh M. The spectrum of nonasthmatic inflammatory airway diseases in adults. *Otolaryngologic Clinics of North America*. 2010;43(1):131–43, ix.

6

Hypersensitivity in chronic cough

Anne E. Vertigan and Peter G. Gibson

The previous chapters described the normal physiology of cough and medical conditions associated with chronic refractory cough. This chapter discusses hypersensitivity in chronic cough. Hypersensitivity relating to cough is a broad concept. Hypersensitivity involves a number of features including cough triggers, central sensitisation and airway hyperresponsiveness, vagal neuropathy, and cough reflex sensitivity.

We define cough hypersensitivity as cough occurring in response to low threshold tussive stimuli, non-tussive stimuli or abnormal laryngeal sensation. It can be measured by cough reflex sensitivity testing and may be centrally or peripherally mediated. We define laryngeal hypersensitivity as cough, paradoxical vocal fold movement, or laryngeal or pharyngeal constriction occurring as a habit or in response to environmental stimuli. It is frequently accompanied by abnormal laryngeal sensation and can be measured using the Laryngeal Hypersensitivity Questionnaire[1] and formal provocation tests.

The traditional view of chronic cough was described by the Anatomic Diagnostic Protocol (Figure 6.1A). This view considered that chronic cough was the outcome of diseases such as asthma, rhinitis and gastroesophageal reflux disease which caused stimulation of the afferent limb of the cough reflex via the vagal nerve. These diseases were believed to be the cause of the cough, and treatment of the associated disease was thought to eliminate cough. More recently, Cough Hypersensitivity Syndrome has been proposed to be the cause of chronic cough (Figure 6.1B). Patients with chronic cough have underlying cough hypersensitivity which is triggered by non-noxious stimuli. Associated diseases such as gastroesophageal reflux disease, or post nasal drip act as triggers or modulators for the cough rather than the underlying cause of the condition.[2]

In recent years there has been discussion of laryngeal hypersensitivity in patients with chronic cough and related laryngeal disorders. The larynx can become hypersensitive whereby there is a low threshold for laryngeal closure.[3] It would appear that both vagal neuropathy and central sensitisation are implicated in chronic refractory cough and laryngeal hypersensitivity syndrome. Therefore, assessment and treatment may need to target both these aspects.

Triggers

Cough triggers are an important component in understanding cough and laryngeal hypersensitivity. Triggers are the first stage in the Urge to Cough model as discussed in Chapter 2. Triggers stimulate the cough receptors and, subsequently, the afferent limb of the cough reflex. Cough triggers are divided into three categories: tussive, non-tussive and paraesthesia.

Tussive triggers

Tussive triggers are those that would normally trigger a cough in healthy individuals. Examples of tussive triggers include smoke, fumes, cigarettes, aspiration, bleach, and noxious aerosols. In patients with chronic refractory cough, however, tussive triggers will trigger a cough at subthreshold levels. For example, while exposure to fumes will trigger cough in most individuals, it will trigger cough at subthreshold doses in patients with chronic cough. Another example is gastroesophageal reflux. Severe reflux into the larynx would trigger laryngeal closure and cough in most individuals. However mild reflux episodes, which are normally occurring physiological events, might trigger cough in patients with chronic cough.

Non-tussive triggers

Non-tussive triggers are those which do not normally trigger cough in a healthy individual. Examples of non-tussive triggers include talking, cold air, perfume, eating, drinking, humidity, air conditioning and exercise. These triggers are commonly reported in many patients with chronic refractory cough. For example, a patient may report coughing in response to perfume, walking inside an air conditioned building, or after talking for an extended period.

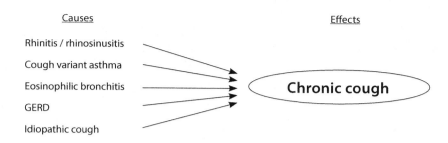

(A) Anatomic diagnostic protocol

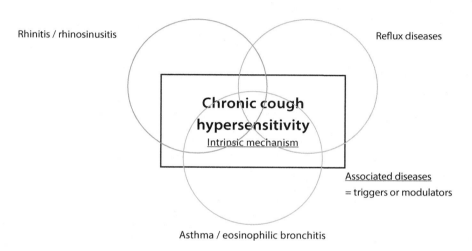

(B) Cough hypersensitivity syndrome

Figure 6.1: Paradigms for chronic cough. **(A)** Anatomic Diagnostic Protocol: cough is considered as the outcome from causative diseases affecting anatomically relevant cough reflex pathways. **(B)** Cough Hypersensitivity Syndrome. Chronic cough hypersensitivity is a common intrinsic mechanism for chronic cough. Commonly associated diseases are triggers or modulators for cough reflex pathways. GERD = gastroesophageal reflux disease. Adapted from Song.[2]

Paraesthesia

Laryngeal paraesthesia includes laryngeal irritability, an abnormal laryngeal sensation and other internal sensations such as an irritation or itch in the throat. These sensations occur in the absence of any external stimuli. Patients with chronic refractory cough may cough in response to a sensation of irritation in the larynx. In fact, this sensation is a trigger for cough in most patients (92%). This finding suggests that laryngeal hypersensitivity is part of the symptom profile of chronic refractory cough. Anecdotally, some patients are as concerned about the abnormal laryngeal sensation as the motor act of coughing.[4]

Trigger frequency and potency

A study of triggers in chronic refractory cough[4] identified the most common triggers as paraesthesia (85%), or non-tussive triggers such as talking (71%), talking on the telephone (56%), and shortness of breath (53%). Exposure to these non-tussive stimuli is often unavoidable. In this study, there was no correlation between the degree of exposure to a particular trigger and the extent to which that trigger resulted in cough. Talking was a significant trigger for cough regardless of the amount of talking. This finding was consistent with our earlier hypothesis that phonation stimulates pressure receptors in the larynx that trigger cough.[5]

Trigger potency was defined as the percentage of patients who cough if exposed to a particular trigger. The most potent cough triggers are fumes, throat irritability and shortness of breath as patients who are exposed to those triggers will frequently cough. However, exposure to these triggers is typically limited, infrequent and often avoidable. Relatively few patients had a solely tussive trigger pattern.[4] Although most patients report coughing following exposure to known tussive stimuli, such as smoke and fumes, most were not exposed to these stimuli, possibly as they have learned to avoid them.

Many patients with chronic cough and voice disorders report an uncomfortable mucous sensation in the throat. Bonhilla[6] reported that mucous results in an uncomfortable sensation which results in the need to cough and throat clear. During mucous clearing, large endolaryngeal contact pressures occur between the arytenoid cartilages and vocal folds. A high percentage of healthy individuals had mucous detected on nasendoscopy (79%) and stroboscopy (97%), although more standardised systems are required to rate mucous.[6] Patients with chronic refractory cough and voice disorders may be more sensitive to normally occurring mucous.

Central sensitisation in chronic cough

Triggers in chronic refractory cough can be characterized and interpreted using a neuropathic framework[7] that provides a role for central sensitisation of the cough reflex. Chronic refractory cough is frequently associated with abnormal laryngeal sensation, consistent with laryngeal paresthesia, and cough is often triggered by stimuli that are considered non-tussive stimuli such as phonation, exercise, and stress/anxiety. In addition, there is also evidence of hypertussia where cough is triggered by low-threshold tussive stimuli. These concepts are the features of sensitization of the cough reflex and are consistent with the concept of chronic refractory cough as a sensory neuropathy.

A further argument for central sensitisation in cough has been described by reinterpreting gastroesophageal reflux and post nasal drip as triggers for cough, rather than a cause of cough.[8] Triggers for cough such as reflux and rhinitis may be innocuous, but have the potential to stimulate vagal afferent nerves. Patients with chronic refractory cough appear to be hypersensitive to internal vagal stimuli such as reflux events.[8] Patients with temporal reflux cough association, where the timing of reflux events and cough events occurs within a one minute window, also have increased cough reflex sensitivity.[9] Therefore, central sensitization might explain neuronal crosstalk between the esophagus and the cough reflex, but also suggests that these patients are sensitised to airway as well as esophageal stimuli.

Patients with chronic refractory cough and related laryngeal disorders have abnormal laryngeal sensation and an overlap in sensory dysfunction during quantitative testing. Sensory testing was performed in patients with a range of laryngeal conditions including chronic refractory cough, paradoxical vocal fold movement, globus pharyngeus and muscle tension dysphonia. Results showed impaired laryngeal sensation in these patient groups compared to healthy controls, but no significant differences between the clinical groups. These findings may suggest a common mechanistic pathway active in these syndromes and might implicate sensory neural dysfunction.[10]

Cross-stimulus responses provide additional support for central sensitization and a common sensory pathway abnormality. Cross-stimulus responses occur when a primary stimulus, such as *phonation*, elicits a sensory response in another domain, such as *cough*. Studies using phonation as the stimulus (Voice Stress Testing, described in more detail in Chapter 8) have shown an increased urge to cough, dyspnea, laryngeal paraesthesia, dysphonia and increased fall in forced inspiratory flow (FIF_{50}). In addition, voice quality has been shown to deteriorate following cough reflex sensitivity testing.[10] In this case, a cough stimulus results in changes to phonation. Hypersensitivity is said to be present, as an increased stimulus in one modality leads to an increased response in another modality. These responses are not triggered by peripheral stimuli, i.e. cough is triggered without a cough stimulus and dysphonia is triggered without a voice stimulus. It is plausible that this process occurs due to central sensitisation.

Chronic pain

Many of the concepts and clinical features that occur in chronic neuropathic pain can be usefully applied to patients with chronic refractory cough and help us to understand the role of central sensitisation in cough. There are a number of similarities between chronic refractory cough and chronic pain, and discussion of these concepts can aid the understanding of the condition.

Neural hypersensitivity is best characterised in chronic pain syndromes. Clinically useful features that allow recognition of a neuropathic pain syndrome are those that indicate sensitization of the pain reflex, such as paresthesia (abnormal sensation), hyperalgesia (pain triggered by a lower level exposure to a known painful stimulus, or increased perception of pain for a given stimulus level), and allodynia (pain triggered by a nonpainful stimulus, such as touch).[7] These features are similar to those occurring in chronic refractory cough and laryngeal symptoms in chronic refractory cough can be reinterpreted in a similar manner.[4] Patients with cough frequently describe symptoms that suggest sensitization of the cough reflex and a neuropathic response. Examples are an abnormal throat sensation, for example, tickle; representing laryngeal paresthesia; increased cough sensitivity in response to a known tussigen, for example, smoke (hypertussia); and cough that is triggered in response to a nontussive stimulus, for example, talking (allotussia). These concepts are summarised in Table 6.1 and examples of the triggers are reported in Table 6.2.

The process of central sensitisation is similar to the development of neuralgia in chronic pain. Neuralgia is pain produced by a change in neurological structure or function. It is non-nociceptive pain, i.e. pain that is not related to activation of pain receptor cells in any part of the body. Damage to the sensory nerves leading

Neuropathic pain			Neuropathic cough		
Concept	*Definition/Description*	*Example*	*Concept*	*Definition/Description*	*Example*
Parasthesia	Abnormal sensation	Tingling sensation in the skin	Laryngeal paraesthesia or hypersensitivity	Abnormal sensation in the throat	Tickle or itch in throat
Hyperalgesia	Increased response to a stimulus that is normally painful but at a reduced threshold	Increased pain response to a needle prick	Hypertussia	Increased cough response to a tussigenic stimulus	Fumes, smoke, aspirate
Allodynia	Pain in response to a stimulus that does not normally produce pain such as a mechanical or thermal stimulus	Pain in response to touch	Allotussia	Cough in response to a non-tussigenic stimulus	Thermal, vocalization, exercise

Table 6.1: Comparison of concepts between chronic refractory cough and neuropathic pain.

81

	Trigger	% Exposed	Tussigenic potency[1]	Relative trigger importance[2]
Laryngeal parasthesia	Sensation/irritability in the throat	94	92	.86
Tussive (hypertussia)	Fumes, bleach, aerosols	40	95	.38
	Smoke	35	78	.27
	Shortness of breath	65	85	.55
Non tussive (allotussia)	Talking, laughing/singing	100	71	.71
	Physical exercise	75	67	.50
	Cold air	52	63	.32
	Stress/anxiety	56	59	.33
	Telephone	100	56	.56
	Eating/drinking	100	48	.48
	Air conditioning	81	45	.36
	Humidity	58	33	.19
	Perfumes	67	29	.19

Table 6.2: Examples of triggers according to chronic pain concepts. Data adapted from *Journal of Voice*, 2011, 25⁵. (1) Trigger potency defined as % triggered if exposed. (2) Relative trigger importance defined as product of % cough if exposed to % exposed.

to axonal degeneration is a possible mechanism for neuralgia.[11] During the subsequent regeneration and healing process, axons from one sensory receptor connect to fibres that previously carried signals from a different sensory receptor. This damage usually starts in unmyelinated fibres of afferent nerves.[11] Increased sensitivity to a painful stimulus may be caused by damage to nociceptors or peripheral nerves.

Laryngeal hypersensitivity is a common feature of neuropathic laryngeal dysfunction. Similarities have been identified between the laryngeal irritability which frequently occurs in chronic refractory cough and neural irritability in trigeminal neuralgia and other neuropathic pain syndromes. We suggest that chronic refractory cough, paradoxical vocal fold movement, globus pharyngeus and some forms of muscle tension dysphonia may be manifestations of laryngeal sensory dysfunction, with a common disturbance of laryngeal function termed laryngeal sensory hyperresponsiveness syndrome. Laryngeal hyperresponsiveness is common regardless of the cause of cough including those with chronic refractory cough.

The similarity between features of chronic refractory cough and chronic pain also suggest a role for central sensitization of the afferent reflex although peripheral sensitization is present in chronic cough.[12] The similar sensory abnormalities between laryngeal dysfunction syndromes also supports the hypothesis of a common neuropathic origin for these syndromes.[10]

Vagal neuropathy

In addition to central sensitisation, chronic cough has also been conceptualised as a form of vagal neuralgia.[13,14] Bastian *et al.*[13] hypothesized that vagal neuralgia could manifest as an exaggerated sensation that is normally mediated by the vagus nerve resulting in a bogus tickle that leads to uncontrollable coughing. In this case, the threshold for initiation of a cough reflex is significantly lowered, and the urge to cough is triggered by low levels of stimuli or even the absence of stimuli. It has been suggested that the sensory threshold of the afferent nerves could be increased following amitriptyline administration thereby inhibiting the cough reflex.[15] Lee and Woo[14] reported recurrent and sensory laryngeal nerve damage in participants with chronic refractory cough, which was subsequently successfully treated with amitriptyline. This study lead the way for subsequent studies into centrally acting neuromodulators in chronic cough such as gabapentin[16] and pregabalin[17] as outlined in Chapter 3.

Airway hyperresponsiveness

Airway hyperresponsiveness refers to an increased sensitivity of the respiratory tract to a variety of pharmacologic and non-pharmacologic stimuli.[18] Hyperresponsiveness can be classified based on the response elicited and the provocation agent used to induce the response. Inhalation of spasmogens such as methacholine and histamine may result in bronchial hyper-responsiveness. Bronchial hyper-responsiveness refers to a narrowing of the intrathoracic or lower airways and is part of the pathophysiology of asthma. In contrast, extrathoracic airway hyperresponsiveness refers to narrowing of the extrathoracic or upper airway. The extrathoracic airways may be hyperresponsive to a variety of stimuli, leading to variable extrathoracic airway obstruction, reflexive glottal spasm and a reduction in inspiratory airflow, whereas functionally, paradoxical movement of the vocal folds is observed.[19,20] Extrathoracic airway hyperresponsiveness characterized by variable extrathoracic airflow obstruction and glottal constriction on inspiration may also occur in paradoxical vocal fold movement.[21]

Hyperresponsiveness of the extrathoracic airway has been confirmed following histamine challenge in 25 out of 40 patients with a history of dyspnea and chronic cough, and it is suggested that hyperresponsiveness of the extrathoracic airway may produce symptoms mimicking bronchial asthma.[19] The authors[19] confirmed the association between glottal constriction and paradoxical vocal fold movement by direct visualisation at nasendoscopy. Bucca et al.[19] concluded that inflammation might be the trigger for the airway hyperresponsiveness and that local reflexes with neural receptors as the sensory pathway might be activated during this process.

Bucca et al.[22] found a high incidence of extrathoracic airway hyperresponsiveness in response to histamine provocation in 67% of patients with cough, and concluded that bronchial and extrathoracic airway hyperresponsiveness were triggered independently of each other and that the extrathoracic airway was the site of the constrictive response. Two studies[23,24] have found that cough following capsaicin inhalation challenge is more prevalent in individuals with symptoms characteristic of paradoxical vocal fold movement, than in those with asthma or normal controls. These findings therefore suggest a link between cough reflex sensitivity and paradoxical vocal fold movement symptoms.

Cough reflex sensitivity

Cough reflex sensitivity could be seen as a form of airway hyperresponsiveness but relates specifically to cough rather than overall respiratory function. Cough reflex sensitivity is heightened in patients with chronic cough and is an important part of the pathophysiology of the condition. Individuals with chronic cough have a sensitised cough reflex[25] whereby cough is evoked by tussive stimuli that are normally subthreshold for initiating the cough reflex (for example: fumes, ammonia, shortness of breath),[26] or by non-tussive stimuli that do not normally trigger cough (for example: talking, laughing, cold air). In other words, cough receptors in chronic cough become more easily stimulated and thus respond more readily to lower levels of stimuli. Repeated coughing continues to irritate the airways and stimulate the cough receptors, further lowering the threshold for continued coughing. Responsiveness of the sensory cough nerves can be affected by the presence of inflammatory mediators in the airway, and is an important pathophysiologic mechanism in non-productive cough.[27] Airway inflammation events are likely to be the cause of increased cough reflex sensitivity. Inflammation affects neural function and thus result in a sensitised cough response.[28]

The dose of capsaicin required to trigger cough in patients with chronic refractory cough is significantly lower, compared to healthy controls which indicates increased cough reflex sensitivity. Interestingly, there is no significant difference in C5 dose between the patients with related laryngeal syndromes such as paradoxical vocal fold movement.[10]

Cough sensitivity to inhaled capsaicin decreases when the specific cause of the cough is successfully treated, but does not change when treatment of the cough is unsuccessful.[27] Cough reflex sensitivity also decreases following speech pathology intervention for chronic refractory cough.[29] Based on this finding, it is hypothesised that suppression of the cough through pharmaceutical or behavioural treatment can lead to reduced cough reflex hypersensitivity.

Patients with chronic refractory cough may also have neuronal hypersensitivity to naturally occurring gaseous reflux.[2] This stimulus, although low intensity and innocuous, provokes irritation which leads to cough.[2] Song[2] suggested that pepsin bile, or low pH in gastric juice causes damage to the epithelium resulting in an inflammatory reaction. Macrophages cause an inflammatory response with neuronal proliferation and upregulation of nociceptors, such as those of the transient receptor potential family.[2]

85

The initial cause of cough may have disappeared but the effect on enhancing cough reflex may be more prolonged.[30] This occurs in the event of transient upper respiratory tract infection or exposure to toxic fumes. Various diseases associated with cough could cause greater stimulation to cough receptors through increased mucous, oedema, and release of tussigenic agents such as bradykinin or neuropeptides. Song[2] further suggested that viruses may induce cough reflex hypersensitivity as a means to disseminate themselves further, as there is upregulation of TRPA1 and TRPV1 receptors during viral infection.[2] Song also described how an oestrogen-TRPV1 association might explain why cough reflex sensitivity is increased in females.

Laryngeal hypersensitivity

Laryngeal hypersensitivity may be affected by neural plasticity. Neural plasticity might affect the way in which the laryngeal motor system reacts to an individual sensation or thought.[31] Stemple described four different ways in which the process of neural plasticity can occur. First, afferent inputs can be withdrawn from the central neurone in response to peripheral nerve injury. Subsequently, new connections are made so that stimulation elicits a different response. This process may be seen in cross-stimulus responses whereby a stimulus of one domain affects the function of another domain. Second, viral illness may attack the central nervous system affecting laryngeal motor control. Third, emotional states can cause hypersensitivity when the larynx is involved in the expression of emotion. Finally, the upper airway may react to specific irritants such as laryngopharyngeal reflux. Stemple[31] claimed that symptoms usually manifest with psychological stressors or postural factors which make the laryngopharynx more susceptible to constriction. Cough hypersensitivity can be due to inflammation which is caused by viral illness and gaseous reflux.

Sensory hyperresponsiveness is a relevant component of the laryngeal dysfunction syndromes. Laryngeal discomfort can suggest the presence of a sensory neuropathic disorder and is present in a range of laryngeal conditions. Patients with chronic refractory cough frequently report irritation and discomfort in the laryngeal region. The common descriptions are of abnormal laryngeal sensation, phlegm, and mucous in the throat, and a tickle or irritation in the throat. However the focus of treatment in these conditions involves motor rather than sensory areas of dysfunction.

It would appear that the laryngeal sensation is similar between patients with a range of laryngeal conditions and may suggest some underlying sensory neuropathy. These findings are consistent with results of quantitative sensory testing in patients with laryngeal sensory hyperresponsiveness syndromes.

Laryngeal hypersensitivity may be related to the laryngeal chemo reflex. This reflex is described by Bucca.[32] In newborns, it results in vocal fold adduction and apnea, whereas adults have cough and airway constriction. It is initiated when nerve receptors in the mucosal epithelial cells of the epiglottis, aryepiglottic folds and interarytenoid space are stimulated. The afferent nerve impulse is carried along the superior laryngeal nerve resulting in an efferent impulse in the recurrent laryngeal nerve which subsequently results in vocal fold adduction. Reflexes become more sensitive with inflammation, viral infection and frequent stimulation from acid and other solutions.

Cough Hypersensitivity Syndrome

Morice proposed the concept of Cough Hypersensitivity Syndrome to explain the pathogenesis of chronic refractory cough.[33] Morice argues that chronic cough should be viewed as a single disorder, i.e. Cough Hypersensitivity Syndrome. This view is in contrast to previous work that identified several subtypes of chronic cough, such as cough due to asthma. Morice believes reflux, either non-acid or gaseous, is the single stimulus for cough hypersensitivity syndrome. Cough Hypersensitivity Syndrome can be used to explain cough due to known causes such as asthma and reflux, but also can replace terms such as chronic idiopathic cough and unexplained cough. Cough Hypersensitivity Syndrome occurs when the initiating cause of cough has disappeared but the enhanced cough reflex remains. It is accompanied by a tickle in the throat. Increased cough reflex sensitivity results from increased sensitivity of cough receptors, plasticity of afferent innervation including nerve density or altered expression of ion channels.[43–45] There is increased expression of TRPV1 in epithelial nerves in non-asthmatic chronic cough. Patients with chronic refractory cough also have inflammation, remodelling in airway submucosa, increased submucosal mast cells, airway wall modelling with goblet cell hyperplasia, subepithelial fibrosis, increased vascularity, and increased mast cells.

One appealing benefit of the Cough Hypersensitivity Syndrome concept is that it provides a useful way of understanding unexplained cough or chronic idiopathic cough. In fact, chronic idiopathic cough has no causative factors[30] and may be better referred to as Cough Hypersensitivity Syndrome. A proportion of patients with unexplained cough have airway sensory hyperreactivity to odorous chemicals and scents, and increased cough reflex sensitivity.[34] Although cough can be due to diseases such as asthma and rhinitis, only a small proportion of patients with these conditions actually cough.[35] Cough Hypersensitivity Syndrome suggests that these etiologies cause cough in the individuals with underlying cough hypersensitivity.[33]

However, while Cough Hypersensitivity Syndrome promises an attractive way of understanding cough, a number of issues need to be addressed before it can become a valid clinical concept. There needs to be a sound definition of Cough Hypersensitivity Syndrome, a clear understanding of the underlying mechanism, reliable measurement that offers diagnostic value, and tools to treat the condition.[35] The specific role of central and peripheral mechanisms in the pathogenesis is yet to be determined.

There needs to be clarification about whether associated laryngeal conditions and symptoms such as paradoxical vocal fold movement and dysphonia are part of the condition of Cough Hypersensitivity Syndrome. Cough Hypersensitivity Syndrome has not been described in related laryngeal conditions, such as muscle tension dysphonia and paradoxical vocal fold movement, and yet these patient groups have increased cough reflex hypersensitivity and increased cough frequency.[10] Furthermore, both the patient experience and objective sensory testing are affected similarly between patients with these related laryngeal conditions. To date, we do not know whether there is any significant clinical difference in patients described as having Cough Hypersensitivity Syndrome and those with combined chronic cough and paradoxical vocal fold movement.

Etiology of hypersensitivity

The syndromes of chronic refractory cough, paradoxical vocal fold movement, globus pharyngeus, and muscle tension dysphonia present to clinicians as discrete and unrelated abnormalities of different aspects of laryngeal motor function; that is, cough, breathing, and phonation.[10] However, these conditions have overlapping symptomatology, and the symptoms are not limited to the domains of cough, respiration and phonation. These conditions also respond similarly to speech pathology intervention. These observations may suggest a common mechanistic pathway such as laryngeal hypersensitivity in these disorders of laryngeal dysfunction.[10]

Occupational exposure

Occupational exposure to irritants can trigger symptoms of chronic refractory cough and paradoxical vocal fold movement. Co-workers may be exposed to the same irritant yet not experience symptoms. Patients experiencing respiratory symptoms might be more susceptible to irritant exposure. A distinction needs to be made between discomfort and damage. These exposures often result in discomfort which is not harmful i.e. the patient has increased sensitivity and lowered thresholds for triggering respiratory symptoms.

Post viral illness

There is often a temporal association between chronic refractory cough and upper respiratory tract infection.[35] Cough is a common symptom associated with upper respiratory tract infection[36] and viral upper respiratory tract infection is a predominant trigger of coughing attacks in both acute and chronic cough.[37] During viral infection, the cough reflex becomes hypersensitive for a limited period of time. Under normal circumstances the cough correspondingly resolves with decreasing cough reflex hypersensitivity. However in some cases, the increased cough reflex sensitivity persists following resolution of viral infection, i.e. longer than three weeks, and leads to persisting cough.[28] In some individuals, cough reflex sensitivity remains elevated even after resolution of the infection. There is evidence that post viral illness may cause hyperresponsiveness that subsequently manifests as chronic cough or paradoxical vocal fold movement, possibly through airway inflammation with or without transient airway hyperresponsiveness.[37] Morrison *et al.*[38] found that viral illness coincided with the onset of cough and paradoxical vocal fold movement in one third of their patients, leading them to speculate that viral illness leads to central nervous system changes. Viruses can affect the peri-aqueductal gray in the brainstem which is an area involved in phonation.[31] These areas become more sensitive to sensory stimuli from the larynx and surrounding structures.[31]

These concepts are consistent with Altman *et al.*[39] and Lee and Woo[14] who proposed that some patients with chronic cough sustained vagal injury from viral infection and that airway hyperresponsiveness might persist beyond the resolution of the acute upper respiratory tract infection. The hyperresponsiveness could manifest as a decrease in the cough threshold in response to irritating stimuli causing patients to be more susceptible to chemical or mechanical stimulation of the cough reflex. Taramarcaz *et al.*[40] described viral respiratory infection as a trigger of paradoxical vocal fold movement. Objectively confirmed viral infection was associated with an exacerbation of paradoxical vocal fold movement in three participants.

Habitual factors

Cough causes repetitive mechanical impact on airway cells.[30] This impact releases chemical mediators which enhance cough through inflammation. In turn, this process causes a positive feed forward system for cough persistence and results in inflammation and tissue remodelling. In short, cough causes increased cough reflex sensitivity which again maintains cough.

Habitual factors can be implicated in the development and maintenance of chronic cough[41] and can contribute to cough occurring in the presence of other causative factors such as asthma and reflux. A habit is a semi-voluntary activity, reinforced either because it is self-soothing or because of the response the activity elicited from the environment.[42] A cough might be stimulated by physical complications of chronic cough such as increased cough reflex sensitivity and maintained by environmental factors.[41] Physical coughing may in turn stimulate irritant receptors in the airway mucosa while persistent irritation and edema of the pharynx and larynx may also increase the urge to cough. Behavioural management of chronic refractory cough can break the cycle of reciprocal irritation of cough receptors when medical intervention has failed, by increasing voluntary control, reducing cough reflex sensitivity, reduced laryngeal irritation though improved vocal hygiene and treatment of coexisting paradoxical vocal fold movement.

Summary

Hypersensitivity is an emerging concept in the field of chronic cough. Evidence for the concept of central sensitisation in chronic cough is similar to chronic pain and includes the response to centrally acting neuromodulators and cross stimulus responses. Cough reflex sensitivity is also impaired in chronic cough. It improves with speech pathology intervention but not with centrally acting neuromodulators. This suggests that cough reflex sensitivity is peripheral and that speech pathology intervention has a peripheral target. Despite these findings there is still much to be learned about the role of hypersensitivity in chronic cough. Although the cerebral cortex has a role in cough, its role in central sensitisation is unclear. The extent to which central sensitisation or vagal neuropathy effect an individual patient is not known. There might be patient subgroups with a predominant central or peripheral sensitivity pattern. If this is the case it would enable more specific treatment to be targeted.

We hypothesise that an initial injury or inflammation to a site with vagal afferent nerve innervation may lead to cough or laryngeal hyperresponsiveness. This inflammation leads to increased cough reflex sensitivity or laryngeal hyper-sensitivity and may lead to changes in peripheral nerve function. The cycle is perpetuated by repeated coughing or laryngeal constriction. Central sensitisation plays a role in cough where stimulation in one area mediated by the vagus nerve causes a response in another area, e.g. stimulation of the esophagus triggering cough. Additional research is needed to determine whether there is individual susceptibility in the development of central sensitisation. Furthermore, while cough reflex sensitivity can be modified with changes to cough behaviour, the extent to which cough behaviour affects central sensitisation is unclear.

References

1. Vertigan AE, Bone SL, Gibson PG. Development and validation of the Newcastle laryngeal hyper-sensitivity questionnaire. *Cough.* 2014;10(1):1.

2. Song W-J, Chang Y-S, Morice A. Changing the paradigm for cough: does 'cough hypersensitivity' aid our understanding? *Asia Pacific Allergy.* 2013;4(1):3–13.

3. Kenn K, Balkissoon R. Vocal cord dysfunction: what do we know? *European Respiratory Journal.* 2011;37:194–200.

4. Vertigan A, Gibson P. Chronic refractory cough as a laryngeal sensory neuropathy: Evidence from a reinterpretation of cough triggers. *Journal of Voice.* 2011;25(5):596–601.

5. Vertigan A, Theodoros D, Winkworth A, Gibson P. Acoustic and electroglottographic voice characteristics in chronic cough and paradoxical vocal fold movement. *Folia Phoniatrica et Logopaedica.* 2008;60(4):210–6.

6. Bonilha H, Aikman A, Hines K, Deliyski D. Vocal fold mucus aggregation in vocally normal speakers. *Logopedics, Phoniatrics, Vocology.* 2008;33(3):136–42.

7. Jensen T, Baron R. Translation of symptoms and signs into mechanisms in neuropathic pain. *Pain.* 2003;102:1–8.

8. Kahrilas P, Smith J, Dicpinigaitis P. A causal relationship between cough and gastroesophageal reflux disease (GERD) has been established: a pro/con debate. *Lung.* 2014;192(1):39–46.

9. Smith JA, Decalmer S, Kelsall A, *et al.* Acoustic cough—reflux associations in chronic cough: potential triggers and mechanisms. *Gastroenterology.* 2010;139(3):754–62.

10. Vertigan AE, Bone SL, Gibson PG. Laryngeal sensory dysfunction in laryngeal hypersensitivity syndrome. *Respirology*. 2013;18(6):948–56.

11. Latremoliere A, Woolf C. Central sensitization: A generator of pain hypersensitivity by central neural plasticity. *Journal of Pain*. 2009;10:895–926.

12. Groneberg DA, Niimi A, Dinh QT, *et al*. Increased expression of transient receptor potential vanilloid-1 in airway nerves of chronic cough. *American Journal of Respiratory & Critical Care Medicine*. 2004;170(12):1276–80.

13. Bastian R, Vaidya A, Delsupehe K. Sensory neuropathic cough: A common and treatable cause. *Otolaryngology Head & Neck Surgery*. 2006;135(1):17–21.

14. Lee B, Woo P. Chronic cough as a sign of laryngeal sensory neuropathy: Diagnosis and treatment. *Annals of Otology, Rhinology & Laryngology*. 2005;114(4):253–7.

15. Jeyakumar A, Brickman TM, Haben M. Effectiveness of amitriptyline versus cough suppressants in the treatment of chronic cough resulting from postviral vagal neuropathy. *The Laryngoscope*. 2006;116(12):2108–12.

16. Ryan N, Birring S, Gibson P. Gabapentin for refractory chronic cough: a randomised, double-blind, placebo-controlled trial. *The Lancet*. 2012;380(9853):1583–9.

17. Halum S, Sycamore D, McRae B. A new treatment option for laryngeal sensory neuropathy. *The Laryngoscope*. 2009;119:1844–7.

18. deMeer G. Airway responsiveness to direct and indirect stimuli: A population based approach. Doctoral thesis, University of Utrecht, The Netherlands 1961.

19. Bucca C, Rolla G, Scappaticci E, *et al*. Histamine hyperresponsiveness of the extrathoracic airway in patients with asthma symptoms. *Allergy*. 1991;46:147–53.

20. Gibson P, Taramarcaz P, Borgas T. Evaluation of diagnostic tests for vocal cord dysfunction. *American Journal of Respiratory and Critical Care Medicine*. 2004;169:A317.

21. Brugman S (ed). Pediatric side of VCD with emergency management. Presented at: *Advances in the Diagnosis and Treatment of Vocal Cord Dysfunction Conference*, National Jewish Medical and Research Center; 2003; Denver, Colorado.

22. Bucca C, Rolla G, Scappaticci E, *et al*. Extrathoracic and intrathoracic airway responsiveness in sinusitis. *Journal of Allergy and Clinical Immunology*. 1995;95(1):52–7.

23. Millqvist E, Bende M, Lowhagen O. Sensory hyperreactivity: A possible mechanism underlying cough and asthma like symptoms. *Allergy*. 1998;53:1208–12.

24. Ternesten-Hasseus E, Farbrot A, Lowhagen O, Millqvist E. Sensitivity to methacholine and capsaicin in patients with unclear respiratory symptoms. *European Journal of Allergy and Clinical Immunology*. 2002;57(6):501–7.

25. Chung K, Widdicome J, Boushey H (eds). *Cough: Causes, Mechanisms and Therapy*. Melbourne: Blackwell Publishing; 2003.

26. Kallarik M, Undem B. Plasticity of vagal afferent fibres mediating cough. In: Chung K, Widdicome J, Boushey H (eds). *Cough: Causes, Mechanisms and Therapy*. Melbourne: Blackwell Publishing; 2003.

27. O'Connell F, Thomas V, Pride N, Fuller R. Cough sensitivity to inhaled capsaicin decreases with successful treatment of chronic cough. *American Journal of Respiratory and Critical Care Medicine*. 1993;150:374–80.

28. McGarvey L, McKeagney P, Polley L, *et al*. Are there clinical features of a sensitized cough reflex? *Pulmonary Pharmacology & Therapeutics*. 2009;22:59–64.

29. Ryan N, Vertigan A, Gibson P. Chronic cough and laryngeal dysfunction improve with specific treatment of cough and paradoxical vocal fold movement. *Cough*. 2009;5(4).

30. Chung K. Chronic 'cough hypersensitivity syndrome': a more precise label for chronic cough. *Pulmonary Pharmacology & Therapeutics*. 2011;24(3):267–71.

31. Stemple J, Fry L. *Voice Therapy: Clinical Case Studies*. 3rd edn. San Diego, CA: Plural Publishing; 2009.

32. Bucca CB, Bugiani M, Culla B. Chronic cough and irritable larynx. *Journal of Allergy and Clinical Immunology*.127(2):412–9.

33. Morice A. The cough hypersensitivity syndrome: A novel paradigm for understanding cough. *Lung*. 2010;188(Suppl 1):S87–S90.

34. Millqvist E. The airway sensory hyperreactivity syndrome. *Pulmonary Pharmacology & Therapeutics*. 2011;24(3):263–6.

35. Morice A, McGarvey L, Dicipinigaitis P. Cough hypersensitivity syndrome is an important clinical concept: a pro/con debate. *Lung*. 2011;190(1):3–9.

36. Hutchings H, Eccles R, Smith A, Jawad M. Voluntary cough suppression as an indication of symptom severity in upper respiratory tract infections. *European Respiratory Journal*. 1993;6:1449–54.

37. Farrer J, Keenan J, Levy P. Understanding the pathology and treatment if virus-induced cough. *Home Healthcare Consultant*. 2001;82(2):10–8.

38. Morrison M, Rammage L, Emami A. The irritable larynx syndrome. *Journal of Voice*. 1999;13(3):447–55.

39. Altman K, Simpson C, Amin M, *et al*. Cough and paradoxical vocal fold motion. *Otolaryngology Head & Neck Surgery*. 2002;127(6):501–11.

40. Taramarcaz P, Grissell T, Borgas T, Gibson P. Transient post-viral vocal cord dysfunction. *Journal of Allergy and Clinical Immunology*. 2004;114(6):1471–2.

41. Pierce R, Watson T. Psychogenic cough in children: A literature review. *Children's Health Care*. 1998;27(1):63–76.

42. Wamboldt M, Wamboldt F. Psychiatric aspects of respiratory symptoms. In: Taussig L, Landau L (eds). *Pediatric Respiratory Medicine*. St Louis, MO: Mosby; 1999.

43. Birring S. Controversies in the evaluation and management of chronic cough. *American Journal of Respiratory & Critical Care Medicine*. 2011;183(6):708–15.

44. Morice A. The cough hypersensitivity syndrome: A novel paradigm for understanding cough. *Lung*. 2010;188(Suppl 1):S87–S90.

45. Chung KF. Approach to chronic cough: the neuropathic basis for cough hypersensitivity syndrome. *Journal of Thoracic Disease*. 2014:S699–S707.

7

Laryngeal dysfunction in chronic cough

Anne E. Vertigan and Peter G. Gibson

In previous years, little consideration was given to the role of the larynx in chronic cough. In fact, many of the anatomical diagrams in the respiratory medicine literature included the lungs, trachea and oral cavity but no larynx! However, we now believe the larynx has an important role in chronic cough. The previous chapter outlined cough and laryngeal hypersensitivity in chronic refractory cough. This chapter will explore the relationship between dysphonia and chronic refractory cough, and describe laryngeal dysfunction syndromes that can be associated with chronic refractory cough.

There are several reasons why the larynx has been implicated in chronic refractory cough. First, it has been found that 50% of patients with cough also have coexisting laryngeal dysfunction that was characterised as paradoxical vocal fold movement on nasendoscopy and pulmonary function testing.[1] Second, patients with chronic refractory cough can have coexisting clinically significant voice disorders.[2] Finally, many patients with chronic refractory cough report that talking is a frequent trigger of cough.[3,4] In this situation, it is hypothesised that that vocal fold adduction occurring during phonation can trigger cough.[3] Although this evidence suggests that laryngeal function is implicated in chronic refractory cough, the precise nature of the laryngeal dysfunction in is still to be determined.

Dysphonia and chronic cough

Patients referred to speech pathologists with chronic refractory cough may have dysphonia but the cough is considered the core problem, with dysphonia often a coexisting or minor symptom. Not all patients with chronic refractory cough will exhibit dysphonia, or if they do it may be mild and not problematic. Nevertheless, the degree of dysphonia warrants some consideration. There is a complex relationship between dysphonia and cough. Dysphonia is a symptom that can co-occur with chronic refractory cough, and yet coughing and throat clearing can be symptoms of hyperfunctional voice disorders.

Dysphonia has been systematically studied in chronic refractory cough using symptom ratings, auditory perceptual voice analysis, acoustic voice assessment and electroglottography. Self-reported voice symptoms were significantly higher in individuals with chronic refractory cough and paradoxical vocal fold movement than in healthy controls.[3] Previous research found that up to 86% of patients with chronic refractory cough have a deviation in perceptual voice quality and that 40% of these are either moderate or severe deviations.[2] The most frequently reported perceptual voice features were breathy, rough, strained and glottal fry vocal qualities, the majority of these ranging from slight to moderate in severity. Auditory perceptual voice characteristics were similar to those found in Muscle Tension Dysphonia but were generally less severe.[2]

Instrumental voice measures such as maximum phonation time, harmonic to noise ratio, phonation frequency range, fundamental frequency in connected speech, jitter, standard deviation of fundamental frequency and duration of closed phase of vocal fold vibration are impaired in individuals with chronic refractory cough compared to healthy controls.[5] In this study, there was a consistent overlap between patients with chronic refractory cough and those with combined chronic refractory cough and paradoxical vocal fold movement on all acoustic and electroglottographic measures. There were also similarities in the vocal features between patients with chronic refractory cough and those with muscle tension dysphonia although patients with chronic refractory cough had lower fundamental frequency, shorter closed phase of vocal fold vibration and lower jitter values than those with muscle tension dysphonia.

A number of physiological correlates to the voice assessment results have been hypothesised from the results of these studies. Subglottal pressure may be reduced in the patients with chronic refractory cough as evidenced by glottal fry, reduced fundamental frequency, reduced phonation frequency range and monotone vocal quality. Reduced vocal fold closure during phonation in patients with chronic refractory cough and paradoxical vocal fold movement has been proposed due to the presence of breathy voice quality, reduced maximum phonation times and reduced closed phase values.[2,4] Talking is a common trigger for cough, which suggests that vocal fold adduction could exacerbate stimulation of the cough receptors and trigger coughing.[3] If this is true, then reduced vocal fold closure could be an unconscious attempt to reduce stimulation of cough receptors during phonation.

Evidence relating to vocal fold tension in chronic refractory cough has been variable. Patients with chronic refractory cough have increased strained vocal quality and increased jitter values suggesting increased vocal fold tension. Increased muscle tension was hypothesised to be a compensatory mechanism occurring in response to increased laryngeal sensitivity. Improvements in breathy and strained voice qualities following speech pathology intervention for chronic refractory cough could be due to reduced vocal fold tension.[6]

A model hypothesising the relationship between dysphonia and cough is proposed in Figure 7.1. This model suggests that there are some similarities in underlying precipitating features between patients with chronic refractory cough and several voice disorders. Dysphonia in individuals with chronic refractory cough can be due to a separate coexisting diagnosis of muscle tension dysphonia, a direct result of associated diagnostic triggers of the cough such as reflux, and increased cough reflex sensitivity, or alternatively, due to the consequences of cough such as vocal fold oedema or abnormal compensatory laryngeal movements.

There is potential for voice problems to be overlooked in chronic refractory cough, particularly as patients with these conditions primarily complain of cough and respiratory symptoms. According to the model outlined in Figure 7.1, there may be individual variability in the etiology of dysphonia in chronic refractory cough Therefore, dysphonia should be examined on an individual basis during the assessment process with specific reference to case history, severity of the auditory perceptual voice analysis, fundamental frequency and closed phase measures. Although individuals with chronic refractory cough might present with voice problems, they are in most cases, primarily concerned about their cough and respiratory symptoms and are relatively less concerned about their voice. Therefore, it is important to determine patients' degree of concern about

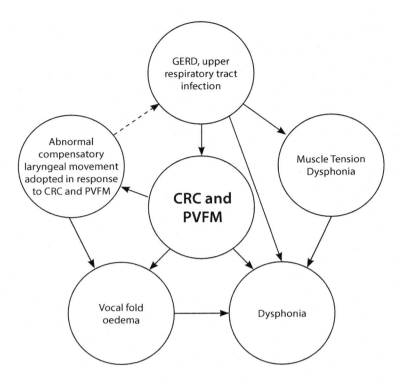

Figure 7.1: Relationship of dysphonia to chronic cough and paradoxical vocal fold movement.

their voice, and establish goals for both voice and cough on an individual basis when developing the treatment plan.

Along with the concept that coughing may exacerbate dysphonia, it is plausible that the reverse may also be true and that the pattern of phonation might contribute to coughing. Vocal hyperfunction and hyperadduction may lead to irritation and stimulation of pressure receptors in the airway and contribute to cough. Scherer *et al.*[7] demonstrated that a vocally fatiguing task consisting of reading loudly from a text at a specified pitch for one hour, resulted in, among other things, a desire to cough in one of their two subjects. This sensation resolved following a period of voice rest. Although this evidence was based on a single case study, it might indicate some interaction between patterns of phonation and the pathogenesis of cough. If this hypothesis were to be confirmed it would have implications for behavioural management of chronic refractory cough, and suggests that speech pathology intervention for chronic refractory cough may need to target phonatory patterns.

Further support for this concept can be inferred from a study where inflammatory mediators were measured before and after a vocally fatiguing task.[8]

In this study, inflammatory mediators increased following a vocally fatiguing task. These mediators decreased following Resonant Voice Therapy, but not after voice rest or habitual talking. Although this was a preliminary study, it demonstrates that airway inflammation can be affected positively and negatively by phonatory patterns. This evidence can be used to shape speech pathology treatment programs.

In order to determine whether the dysphonia is a coexisting or separate condition, voice changes following successful medical or behavioural treatment of cough in an individual case might help to delineate whether or not dysphonia is a secondary side effect of the chronic refractory cough, or evidence of a separate coexisting condition such as muscle tension dypshonia. If voice symptoms resolve following cough treatment, they may have been integral to the cough. Alternatively, if voice symptoms do not resolve following intervention, a separate condition might be present and specific therapy targeting that condition is required.

There is mixed evidence regarding improved vocal fold closure following speech pathology intervention for chronic refractory cough. Improved maximum phonation time and reduced auditory perceptual ratings of breathy vocal quality have been reported following treatment, which may suggest improved vocal fold closure.[6] In contrast, there was no significant change in closed phase values following intervention, a finding that is inconsistent with an improvement in vocal fold closure.[6]

Although chronic refractory cough is considered an entity within respiratory medicine, coughing and throat clearing might be conceptualised differently in the fields of otolaryngology and speech pathology. In some voice disorders, such as vocal nodules and muscle tension dysphonia, coughing and throat clearing are considered phonotraumatic behaviours that have contributed to, exacerbated or perpetuated the voice disorder.[9] These behaviours are considered habitual and are the targets of many treatment programs for voice disorders.[10–12] Coughing and throat clearing cause tissue irritation, alter the biomechanical properties of the vocal fold cover, hinder the regularity of vocal fold vibration, increase irregularities in voice signals, and thus worsen the symptoms of dysphonia.[9,13] Individuals with voice disorders may also exhibit a prolonged cough, but will identify their problem as primarily a voice disorder rather than one of chronic refractory cough. Although dysphonia is the primary complaint, it may be exacerbated by chronic coughing and throat clearing.[9,14] The process can become self-generating as individuals continue to cough in order to relieve the irritation in the throat.[14]

Some individuals with voice disorders will cough or clear their throat deliberately in order to initiate phonation. It is more likely to occur when the individual has difficulty with consistent phonation onset. This behaviour may be easier to target in individuals with voice disorders than in those with chronic refractory cough, by using simple cues to replace the throat clearing behaviour with sipping water or swallowing.

Laryngeal disorders associated with cough

Several laryngeal disorders, such as paradoxical vocal fold movement, muscle tension dysphonia, globus pharyngeus and laryngospasm, have been associated with chronic refractory cough. These disorders often occur in isolation but can co-occur with chronic refractory cough. There is also a similarity in the symptoms and underlying etiologies between these conditions. Awareness of the possibility of these conditions provides a more comprehensive assessment of the patient and enables the appropriate therapy to be targeted to the individual symptom profile. These conditions are described briefly below and the management of paradoxical vocal fold movement and globus pharyngeus is outlined in more detail in Chapters 11 and 12.

Paradoxical vocal fold movement

Paradoxical vocal fold movement (PVFM), also known as vocal cord dysfunction, is a syndrome whereby the vocal folds adduct abruptly, involuntarily and episodically during inspiration leading to symptoms of dyspnea, stridor, dysphonia and cough. This adductor pattern is in contrast to the normal cycle of respiration, whereby the vocal folds abduct slightly during inspiration[15] and adduct slightly during expiration.[16] Closure patterns in paradoxical vocal fold movement are highly variable. Closure may occur on inspiration but there may be an expiratory component.[17] Laryngeal opening during expiration is variable between individuals.[18]

Symptoms of paradoxical vocal fold movement are usually episodic and are localised to the larynx.[19] These symptoms can be categorized as respiratory (dyspnea stridor, cough, wheeze, shortness of breath and air hunger), voice and upper airway (choking, tightness in the neck muscles, throat irritation, sensation of constriction in the larynx and a dry throat). Symptoms in paradoxical vocal fold movement can range from mild breathing discomfort to severe respiratory distress.[18] Acute episodes of paradoxical vocal fold movement can be extremely frightening, and in some cases lead to panic and anxiety.

In people with paradoxical vocal fold movement an obstruction is demonstrated by reduced inspiratory curves on pulmonary function testing and symptomatically, inspiration is noted to be affected more than expiration. There is often pronounced variability in spirometric tests.[20] It does not result in hypoxemia and oxygen saturation during an attack remains normal.[21] The diagnosis of paradoxical vocal fold movement may be suggested when severity of dyspnea appears out of proportion to laboratory findings, and when there is no response to aggressive asthma therapy.[22] Other causes of upper airway obstruction such as granuloma, vocal fold paralysis, subglottic stenosis, tracheomalacia, and laryngomalacia have been excluded during the medical evaluation.[26]

Hicks *et al* described several laryngeal sensory receptors that might be involved in paradoxical vocal fold movement.[18] These include:

1. Cold receptors which respond to changes in temperature
2. Irritant receptors which respond to mechanical stimulation, and to irritants including water and aerosols. These receptors are mostly responsible for the glottal closure reflex.
3. Pressure receptors which respond to changes in laryngeal transmural pressure
4. Drive receptors which respond to laryngeal movement.

Exercise induced paradoxical vocal fold movement is a subtype of paradoxical vocal fold movement. Patients have paradoxical vocal fold movement primarily triggered by intense physical exercise. Dyspnea is seldom present at other times. Patients in this subgroup are typically young, high achieving athletes. Speech pathology intervention can help gain voluntary control over symptoms during exercise, and teach patients to identify and prevent paradoxical vocal fold movement episodes.

Triggers for paradoxical vocal fold movement include upper respiratory tract infection, occupational exposure, physical exertion, coughing, and air pollution.[18] Patients may have a single initiating trigger but then find that symptoms are triggered by a range of triggers that previously were not problematic. Hicks[18] suggests that this is a priming effect. The psychological effects of paradoxical vocal fold movement might be more problematic when the condition goes unrecognised or untreated.

There are a number of similarities between chronic refractory cough and paradoxical vocal fold movement, including medical etiologies, triggers, symptoms, abnormalities of laryngeal function, psychological factors and behavioural treatment strategies.[23–25] These features are outlined in Table 7.1. Many patients present with symptoms suggestive of both chronic refractory cough and paradoxical vocal fold movement. Further, on specific testing, persons who primarily complain of cough have attenuation of the inspiratory curve, which may suggest paradoxical vocal fold movement. Milgrom *et al.*[26] reported that 20% of their patients with chronic cough also had abnormal vocal fold motion on fiberoptic laryngoscopy. The authors claimed that those patients benefited from breathing exercises similar to those developed for the treatment of paradoxical vocal fold movement.

Early literature described chronic refractory cough and paradoxical vocal fold movement as discrete entities and, in clinical practice, they often occur as isolated conditions. The relationship between the conditions may be viewed from a number of perspectives. One perspective is that cough is frequently reported as a symptom of paradoxical vocal fold movement.[27] Objective cough counting using the Leicester Cough Monitor has shown that the number of coughs per hour was actually higher in patients with chronic refractory cough, paradoxical vocal fold movement and muscle tension dysphonia, compared to controls ($p = 0.002$).[28]

Another perspective is that there may be a causal relationship between the conditions, with paradoxical vocal fold movement causing chronic refractory cough.[29] Blager[30] hypothesised that individuals subconsciously cough during an episode of paradoxical vocal fold movement in attempt to relieve vocal fold adduction and maintain airway patency. This theory is consistent with the finding that some patients deliberately cough to relieve an abnormal sensation from their throat.[3] This sensation might be vocal fold adduction occurring during an episode of paradoxical vocal fold movement.

Further evidence for a relationship between chronic cough and paradoxical vocal fold movement was provided by Lee and Woo,[31] who found a high prevalence of sensory neuropathy of the recurrent and superior laryngeal nerves in patients with symptoms of chronic cough and laryngospasm. A trial of gabapentin was effective in relieving the laryngeal irritation and cough in these patients.

Features	CRC	PVFM
Associated Symptoms		
Cough	✓	✓
Dysphonia	✓	✓
Globus	✓	✓
Dyspnea	✗	✓
Associated medical conditions		
Asthma	✓	✓
Gastroesophageal reflux	✓	✓
ACE inhibitor use	✓	✓
Rhinosinusitis	✓	✓
Post viral	✓	✓
Other features		
Psychological issues	✓	✓
Implications for quality of life	✓	✓
Exercise induced	✗	✓
Laryngeal hypersensitivity	✓	✓
Intervention		
Refractory to medical treatment	✓	✓
Responds to breathing exercises	✓	✓
Responds to psychological approaches	✓	✗
Responds to behavioural treatment	✓	✓
Diagnosis		
Anatomic diagnostic protocol	✓	✗
Nasendoscopy	✗	✓
Flow volume loop	✓	✓
CT scan	✗	✓

Table 7.1: Comparison of Chronic Refractory Cough and Paradoxical Vocal Fold Movement. ✓ = feature present; ✗ = feature absent; ACE = angiotensin converting enzyme.

103

Support for a link between chronic cough and paradoxical vocal fold movement can also be inferred from Rolla et al.,[32] who studied 14 patients with gastroesophageal reflux disease, seven with cough, and seven without cough. Rolla et al. found that patients with cough had significantly higher upper airway hyperresponsiveness than those without cough.

Altman et al.[33] proposed that paradoxical vocal fold movement along with gastroesophageal reflux disease and vagal neuropathy were causes of cough. The authors suggested that chronic coughing might actually trigger episodes of paradoxical vocal fold movement. Altman et al. hypothesized a mechanism linking chronic cough and paradoxical vocal fold movement, whereby chronic coughing and throat clearing cause chronic irritation to the larynx which, along with other irritants such as gastroesophageal reflux disease and allergens, predispose the larynx to be sensitive to external stimuli that trigger paradoxical vocal fold movement attacks. There is also increased laryngeal hypersensitivity in both conditions which is not readily distinguished.

A model depicting a proposed relationship between chronic cough and paradoxical vocal fold movement is shown in Figure 7.2. This model demonstrates that chronic cough and paradoxical vocal fold movement may be seen on a continuum, with pure chronic cough at one end, pure paradoxical vocal fold movement at the other end, and a combination of features in the middle. A number of underlying etiologies such as gastroesophageal reflux disease might contribute to these two conditions. The two conditions may manifest in a range of clinical signs and symptoms such as cough, dyspnea and dysphonia. We suggest that paradoxical vocal fold movement should be part of the diagnostic paradigm for chronic refractory cough.

There is similarity in the medical conditions associated with chronic refractory cough and paradoxical vocal fold movement, including asthma, gastroesophageal reflux disease and rhinosinusitis. To add to the complexity, however, chronic refractory cough and paradoxical vocal fold movement do not always result from these medical conditions. It has been recently hypothesized that these conditions trigger cough and paradoxical vocal fold movement in vulnerable patients with increased laryngeal hypersensitivity. This assumption would explain why only a subset of patients with these medical conditions, develop chronic cough.

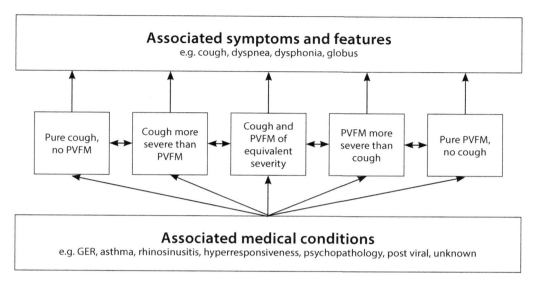

Figure 7.2: Relationship between chronic cough and paradoxical vocal fold movement. Continuum of symptoms in CC and PVFM with pure CC at one end, pure PVFM at the other and a range of symptoms in the middle. There are a number of common etiologies such as GER or rhinosinusitis for these conditions. These conditions result in a number of overlapping symptoms and features including dyspnea, cough, and dysphonia (from *Journal of Voice*).[34]

Laryngospasm

Laryngospasm is distinct from paradoxical vocal fold movement. It is defined as severe and sudden complete vocal fold closure following direct laryngeal stimulation often of noxious stimuli.[35–37] Vocal fold closure is sustained during both inspiration and expiration. This closure is sustained even after removal of noxious stimuli. In contrast, paradoxical vocal fold movement is temporary and resolves after noxious stimuli are removed. Laryngospasm can also occur at night and be triggered by reflux. Laryngospasm and paradoxical vocal fold movement have similar triggers, although paradoxical vocal fold movement can also be triggered by irritants that do not stimulate the larynx.[38] Laryngospasm can be triggered by noxious substances such as ammonia, chlorine, and sulphur dioxide however patients usually have a predisposition.

Despite these distinctions, there is some confusion around terminology. Some clinicians do not make a distinction between laryngospasm and paradoxical vocal fold movement. Murry[35] questioned whether laryngospasm is in fact a severe episode of paradoxical vocal fold movement.

Exercise induced laryngeal obstruction

Nielsen and colleagues[39] have described a condition they term Exercise Induced Laryngeal Obstruction (EILO). EILO is a broad term encompassing exercise induced laryngomalacia, laryngochalasia and paradoxical vocal fold movement and is predominantly described in athletes. The severity of EILO can range from mild to severe where there is complete obstruction of the laryngeal inlet. The study examined athletes, defined as people who exercise for a minimum of ten hours a week, who had been referred for respiratory problems and suspected asthma. Of these patients, 62% had received asthma medication with no objective evidence of airway hyperresponsiveness. The athletes were examined using continuous laryngoscopy during intense exercise while running on a treadmill. Obstruction occurred at either the supraglottic or the vocal fold level and symptoms disappeared once the exercise ceased. In this study, one third of the athletes had EILO, with 10% affecting the vocal folds, 71% affecting the supraglottic area and 19% combined.

Surgical treatment involving removal of the cuniform cartilages has been reported to be successful. EILO has predominantly been reported in European countries, while in other countries it has not been readily distinguished from paradoxical vocal fold movement. Further research examining the difference between these conditions will expand our understanding and may offer new treatment approaches.

Irritable larynx syndrome

Irritable larynx syndrome is a term used to describe a collection of upper airway symptoms including chronic cough, paradoxical vocal fold movement, globus and dysphonia.[24] Irritable larynx syndrome is unlikely to be a separate condition, but rather a term encompassing a collection of related laryngeal conditions. There are slightly different interpretations of this concept in the literature. Morrison *et al.*[24] hypothesised a mechanism linking chronic refractory cough and paradoxical vocal fold movement, in which features such as cough, dysphagia, globus, paradoxical vocal fold movement and muscle tension dysphonia were conceptualised as a subset of hyperfunctional laryngeal symptoms. Sandage and Schroth[40] proposed a continuum of symptoms comprising the irritable larynx syndrome, from throat clearing to chronic cough, then paradoxical vocal fold movement and, finally, laryngospasm. In contrast to Morrison *et al.*,[24] this model did not include dysphonia or laryngeal hyperfunction. Despite the similar terms used, the model proposed by Sandage would appear to be a variation on the original description of the irritable larynx syndrome proposed by Morrison *et al.*

It has been postulated that irritable larynx syndrome, a condition encompassing both chronic cough and paradoxical vocal fold movement, develops as a reaction to central nervous system change, and that this change results in hyperexcitability of sensorimotor pathways and an alteration in the way that central neurones react to incoming stimuli.[24] Irritable larynx syndrome involves plastic change to brainstem laryngeal controlling neuronal networks, through which etiologies such as reflux, psychological problems, habitual postural muscle misuse and central nervous system viral illness can trigger episodes. The sensitivity threshold for the cough behaviour is thought to be remapped in the brain in this condition.[24] In irritable larynx syndrome, the brainstem control of sensory motor programs is altered, resulting in abnormal muscle tension or spasm in response to normal levels of stimulation.[37]

Occupational or work-associated irritable larynx syndrome has also been described.[41] This condition may be triggered by strong odours or irritants. Hoy[41] compared patients with work-associated irritable larynx syndrome and occupational asthma using a chart review. The condition is defined as episodic symptoms associated with a specific triggering stimulus at the workplace. Although not stated by Hoy, it is possible that this condition could also be associated with irritant exposure in any environment.

Diagnostic criteria for work-associated irritable larynx syndrome include episodic symptoms attributable to laryngeal and/or supraglottic tension, presence of a workplace sensory trigger and confirmation of laryngeal tension and exclusion of organic laryngeal pathology. Symptoms include muscular tension dysphonia, dyspnea with sensation of airflow limitation at the level of the throat, globus sensation and chronic cough. Triggers included odours, fumes, perfumes and cleaning agents.

Reactive Airway Dysfunction Syndrome

Reactive Airway Dysfunction Syndrome (RADS) results in cough, chest tightness, wheeze, and shortness of breath within 24 to 72 hours of exposure to a noxious irritant. It was reported in the 9/11 World Trade Centre responders.[42] Key factors in RADS include bronchial hyperresponsiveness and airflow obstruction, and paradoxical vocal fold movement may also be present. There is a significant overlap in the profile of RADS and irritant induced paradoxical vocal

107

fold movement. Cough is also a problematic feature of the condition. The speech pathology assessment and treatment of RADS is similar to that used in chronic cough and paradoxical vocal fold movement.[42]

Summary

Laryngeal conditions are common in patients with chronic refractory cough. There is a complex relationship between chronic cough, paradoxical vocal fold movement, and dysphonia with similarities between the conditions of chronic refractory cough, paradoxical vocal fold movement, globus pharyngeus, and muscle tension dysphonia. These conditions may be part of a single underlying laryngeal sensory hyperresponsiveness syndrome.

References

1. Ryan N, Gibson P. Characterization of laryngeal dysfunction in chronic persistent cough. *The Laryngoscope*. 2009;119:640–645.

2. Vertigan AE, Theodoros DG, Winkworth AL, Gibson PG. Perceptual voice characteristics in chronic cough and paradoxical vocal fold movement. *Folia Phoniatrica et Logopaedica*. 2007;59(5):256–67.

3. Vertigan A, Theodoros D, Gibson P, Winkworth A. Voice and upper airway symptoms in people with chronic cough and paradoxical vocal fold movement. *Journal of Voice*. 2007;21(3):361–83.

4. Vertigan A, Gibson P. Chronic refractory cough as a laryngeal sensory neuropathy: Evidence from a reinterpretation of cough triggers. *Journal of Voice*. 2011;25(5):596–601.

5. Vertigan A, Theodoros D, Winkworth A, Gibson P. Acoustic and electroglottographic voice characteristics in chronic cough and paradoxical vocal fold movement. *Folia Phoniatrica et Logopaedica*. 2008;60(4):210–6.

6. Vertigan AE, Theodoros DG, Winkworth AL, Gibson PG. A comparison of two approaches to the treatment of chronic cough: Perceptual, acoustic, and electroglottographic outcomes. *Journal of Voice*. 2008;22(5):581–9.

7. Scherer R, Titze I, Raphael B, *et al*. Vocal fatigue in a trained and an untrained voice user. In: Baer T, Sasaki C, Harris K (eds). *Laryngeal Function in Phonation and Respiration*. Boston, MA: College Hill Press; 1987.

8. Verdolini Abbott K, Li NYK, Branski R, *et al*. Vocal exercise may attenuate acute vocal fold inflammation. *Journal of Voice*. 2012;26(6):814.e1–.e13.

9. Colton J, Casper J, Leonard R. *Understanding Voice Problems: A Physiological Perspective for Diagnosis and Treatment*. 4th edn. Baltimore, MD: Lippincott Williams & Wilkins; 2011.

10. Ward P, Zwitman D, Hanson D, Berci G. Contact ulcers and granulomas of the larynx: new insights into their etiology as a basis for more rational treatment. *Otolaryngology Head & Neck Surgery*. 1980;88(3):262–9.

11. Ward P, Berci G. Observations on the pathogenesis of chronic non-specific pharyngitis and laryngitis. *The Laryngoscope*. 1982;92(12):1377–82.

12. Broaddus-Lawrence P, Treole K, McCabe R, *et al*. The effects of preventive vocal hygiene education on the habits and perceptual vocal characteristics of training singers. *Journal of Voice*. 2000;14(1):68–71.

13. Hsiao T, Liu C, Hsu C, Lin K. Vocal fold abnormalities in laryngeal tension-fatigue syndromes. *Journal of the Formosan Medical Association*. 2001;100(12):837–40.

14. Boone D, McFarlane S, VonBerg S, Zraick R. *The Voice and Voice Therapy*. 8th edn. Sydney: Allyn & Bacon; 2009.

15. Jamilla F, Stevens D, Szidon P. Vocal cord dysfunction. *Clinical Pulmonary Medicine*. 2000;7(3):111–9.

16. Koufman J. The differential diagnosis of paradoxical vocal cord movement. *The Visible Voice*. 1994;3(3).

17. Balkissoon R, Kenn K. Asthma: Vocal cord dysfunction (VCD) and other dysfunctional breathing disorders. *Seminars in Respiratory and Critical Care Medicine*. 2012;33(6):595–605.

18. Hicks M, Brugman S, Katial R. Vocal cord dysfunction/Paradoxical vocal fold motion. *Primary Care: Clinics in Office Practice*. 2008;35:81–103.

19. Benninger C, Parsons J, Mastronarde J. Vocal cord dysfunction and asthma. *Current Opinion in Pulmonary Medicine*. 2011;17(1):45–9.

20. Perkner J, Fennelly K, Balkissoon R, *et al*. Irritant-associated vocal cord dysfunction. *Journal of Occupational and Environmental Medicine*. 1998;40(2):136–43.

21. Brugman S (ed). Pediatric side of VCD with emergency management. Presented at: *Advances in the Diagnosis and Treatment of Vocal Cord Dysfunction Conference*, National Jewish Medical and Research Center; 2003; Denver, Colorado.

22. Marsh C, Trudeau M, Weiland J. Recurrent asthma despite corticosteroid therapy in a 35 year old woman. *Chest*. 1994;105:1855–7.

23. Bucca C, Rolla G, Scappaticci E, *et al*. Histamine hyperresponsiveness of the extrathoracic airway in patients with asthma symptoms. *Allergy*. 1991;46:147–53.

24. Morrison M, Rammage L, Emami A. The irritable larynx syndrome. *Journal of Voice*. 1999;13(3):447–55.

25. Andrianopoulous M, Gallivan G, Gallivan K. PVCM, PVCD, EPL and Irritable Larynx Syndrome: What are we talking about and how do we treat it? *Journal of Voice*. 2000;14(4):607–18.

26. Milgrom H, Corsello P, Freedman M, *et al*. Differential diagnosis and management of chronic cough. *Comprehensive Therapy*. 1990;16(10):46–53.

27. Brugman S. What's this thing called vocal cord dysfunction? Primary and Critical Care Update. 2006;20(26).

28. Vertigan AE, Bone SL, Gibson PG. Laryngeal sensory dysfunction in laryngeal hypersensitivity syndrome. *Respirology*. 2013;18(6):948–56.

29. Prakash U. Uncommon causes of cough: American College of Chest Physicians Evidence Based Clinical Practice Guidelines. *Chest*. 2006;129(1):206–19.

30. Blager F. Paradoxical vocal fold movement: Diagnosis and management. *Current Opinion in Otolaryngology & Head and Neck Surgery*. 2000;8:180–3.

31. Lee B, Woo P. Chronic cough as a sign of laryngeal sensory neuropathy: Diagnosis and treatment. *Annals of Otology, Rhinology & Laryngology*. 2005;114(4):253–7.

32. Rolla G, Colagrande P, Magnano M, *et al*. Extrathoracic airway dysfunction in cough associated with gastroesophageal reflux. *Journal of Allergy and Clinical Immunology*. 1998;120(1):1–11.

33. Altman K, Simpson C, Amin M, *et al*. Cough and paradoxical vocal fold motion. *Otolaryngology Head & Neck Surgery*. 2002;127(6):501–11.

34. Vertigan AE, Theodoros DG, Gibson PG, Winkworth AL. The relationship between chronic cough and paradoxical vocal fold movement: a review of the literature. *Journal of Voice*. 2006;20(3):466–80.

35. Murry T, Sapienza C. The role of voice therapy in the management of paradoxical vocal fold motion, chronic cough and laryngospasm. *Otolaryngology Clinics of North America*. 2010;43:73–83.

36. Poelmans J, Tack J, Feenstra L. Cough and paradoxical vocal fold motion. *Otolaryngology Head & Neck Surgery*. 2004;49:1868–74.

37. Stemple J, Fry L. *Voice Therapy: Clinical Case Studies*. 3rd edn. San Diego, CA: Plural Publishing; 2009.

38. Kenn K, Balkissoon R. Vocal cord dysfunction: What do we know? *European Respiratory Journal*. 2011;37:194–200.

39. Nielsen E, Hull J, Backer V. High prevalence of exercise-induced larygneal obstruction in athletes. *Medicine and Science in Sports and Exercise*. 2013;45(11):2030–5.

40. Sandage M, Schroth M. Sniffs, gasps and cough: Irritable larynx syndrome. ASHA convention short course: Retrieved February 20, 2006 from http://www.asha.org/about/events/convention/05-archive/program-courses/short_course05.htm; 2005.

41. Hoy RF, Ribeiro M, Anderson J, Tarlo SM. Work-associated irritable larynx syndrome. *Occupational Medicine*. 2010;60(7):546–51.

42. McCabe D, Altman K. Laryngeal hypersensitivity in the World Trade Centre-exposed population. *American Journal of Respiratory & Critical Care Medicine*. 2012;186(5):402–3.

8

Speech pathology assessment of chronic refractory cough

Anne E. Vertigan

The previous chapters have described the characteristics, etiology, and physiology of chronic refractory cough and the medical management of the condition. The following chapters describe speech pathology management of chronic refractory cough. This chapter outlines the assessment process for the speech pathologist including selecting the appropriate patients for treatment, case history interview and assessment procedures.

Referral criteria

The referral process for patients with chronic refractory cough is important as not all patients with chronic cough require speech pathology intervention. Referrals for patients with chronic refractory cough may be influenced by the policy of the service and are likely to vary from country to country. Patients with chronic refractory cough should receive a comprehensive medical evaluation before being referred for speech pathology treatment.[1-3] There is no evidence to support speech pathology treatment of chronic refractory cough prior to medical intervention.[4] Speech pathology treatment should be coordinated with medical management rather than operate in isolation or competition. It should be conceptualised as an adjunct rather than an alternative to medical treatment. Medical intervention, for example treatment for asthma or gastroesophageal reflux disease (GERD), might continue for the duration of the speech pathology treatment in some individuals.

Determining what constitutes appropriate medical management for chronic refractory cough is complex. Medical treatment according to the Anatomic Diagnostic Protocol, whereby known causes of cough such as asthma, rhinosinusitis and gastroesophageal reflux disease are considered and treated, should be a minimum standard. Medical investigation needs to be targeted and not overly excessive. Overly aggressive investigations, can foster the sick role, lead patients to expect a definitive medical explanation,[5] and reduce patient's ability to internalise responsibility for behavioural treatment.

Referral policies for chronic refractory cough and paradoxical vocal fold movement are particularly important for speech pathologists working in settings that allow patients to self-refer. We argue that patients should meet specific referral criteria before being referred for speech pathology intervention. Indicators for referral of individuals with chronic refractory cough to speech pathologists are suggested in Table 8.1. Patients should meet the inclusion criteria prior to being referred for speech pathology intervention. If the cough has persisted for less than two months, or is not problematic for the patient then a speech pathology referral may not be required.

Indicators for referral (Table 8.1) may suggest the presence of related laryngeal conditions that also require speech pathology intervention. For example, inspiratory dyspnea, audible inspiration, or attenuation of the inspiratory limb of the flow volume loop are possible signs of paradoxical vocal fold movement. Glottal constriction during nasendoscopy may be a sign of paradoxical vocal fold movement, or of other hyperfunctional voice disorders. Cough that persists despite a trial of medical treatment for asthma, rhinitis or gastroesophageal reflux disease is likely to be chronic refractory cough and may benefit from speech pathology treatment.

Patients demonstrating any of the exclusion criteria listed in Table 8.1 are not appropriate for speech pathology treatment. These patients may require additional medical investigation and treatment prior to undergoing speech pathology assessment or treatment. In fact, some of these patients may not even require speech pathology intervention. First, if patients have not been reviewed by a respiratory physician or otolaryngologist, then speech pathology intervention may not be appropriate. Specialist medical examination is required to rule out serious medical disease such as tuberculosis or carcinoma, and less serious but treatable associated diseases may need to be managed. Second, speech pathology referral is not appropriate if patients have not undergone spirometry. In

---

Inclusion criteria

Chronic refractory cough

Cough persists for two months following medical treatment

Cough is problematic for the patient

Indicators for referral

Inspiratory dyspnea or audible inspiration

Attenuation of inspiratory limb of flow volume loop during spirometry or provocation challenge

Glottal constriction during inspiration directly observed during nasendoscopy

Dysphonia

Cough persisting despite medical treatment for asthma, gastroesophageal reflux disease and rhinosinusitis

Exclusion criteria

Patient not reviewed by a respiratory physician or otolaryngologist

Spirometry not conducted

Trial of withdrawal of ACE inhibitor not considered by medical practitioner

Untreated gastroesophageal reflux

Untreated asthma

Asthma not reviewed in last two years

Untreated rhinosinusitis

Current upper respiratory tract infection

Table 8.1: Criteria for referral for speech pathology treatment of chronic refractory cough and paradoxical vocal fold movement.

most cases, spirometry is conducted as part of the respiratory medicine review. Spirometry will identify important information that can signal airway disease other than that which is managed by the speech pathologist. Certain classes of medications known as Angiotensin Converting Enzyme Inhibitors (ACE-I), used to treat hypertension, are known to increase cough reflex sensitivity in some individuals. Thus, medical treatment for cough associated with ACE inhibitor use may involve a trial of withdrawing ACE inhibitors, even if there is no temporal association between the onset of cough and commencing medication. This withdrawal needs to be supervised by a medical professional. It must be emphasised that it is beyond the scope of speech pathology practice to provide advice regarding medications. Care should be taken to avoid even mentioning changes to medication directly to patients, in order to avoid patients inadvertently misinterpreting the message as a recommendation to cease taking their medication. Patients with untreated asthma, rhinosinusitis, or gastroesophageal reflux disease may require a trial of medical treatment before referring to speech pathology. The reason for this trial is twofold. First, it may pose a risk to the patient to have an underlying disease such as asthma untreated or under treated. Second, failure to treat the underlying disease may pose a low risk, but provide less than optimal medical care. Patients with both chronic refractory cough and asthma may require a formal review of their asthma to monitor the extent of the disease, ensure optimal medical management, and remove any unnecessary medication.

Speech pathologists may be pressured by patients and referrers to see patients without adequate medical investigation and diagnosis. However, it is recommended that referrals should only be accepted once patients meet the specific criteria for referral.

Some patients with chronic refractory cough are mystified regarding the reason for a referral to speech pathology[6] as they do not have a problem with their speech. These patients require explanation and reassurance that speech pathology is a specific treatment for their disorder, otherwise they may feel their condition has not been appropriately addressed and continue to seek further medications.[1] In order to optimise adherence and motivation with speech pathology intervention it is important for patients to understand the rationale for their referral to speech pathology.[4]

Speech pathology treatment for cough due to current upper respiratory tract infection has not been investigated in the literature. The majority of patients with acute cough arising from an upper respiratory tract infection will resolve spontaneously and therefore not require speech pathology treatment. This argument is certainly valid from a resource allocation perspective. However given that the majority of patients with chronic refractory cough cite the onset of their cough coincides with an upper respiratory tract infection, speech pathologists could have a role in managing acute cough with upper respiratory tract infection, in order to reduce the likelihood of development into chronic refractory cough. This theory is speculative and further research into this area is needed.

Case history interview

The case history interview is the first component of the speech pathology assessment. In addition to providing the speech pathologist with valuable information, participation in the case history interview can improve the patient's insight into their cough. Case history information can be obtained directly from the patient, patient questionnaires, and the medical record. Some aspects of the case history will have been provided by the referring physician and may not need to be collected directly from the patient during the interview. These questionnaires also provide structure that assists patients to report their symptoms. A protocol for collecting the case history information is recorded in Appendix 1 and the detail is explained in the following sections.

Presenting problem

It is important to understand the presenting problem and major symptoms from the patient's perspective. The patient's description of their condition may differ from that provided by their referring doctor. Many patients referred for chronic refractory cough have a wide ranging set of symptoms affecting voice, swallowing and breathing. This broad spectrum of symptoms can make it challenging for the speech pathologist to draw a single conclusion. Broad questions about symptoms are raised early on in the assessment in order to identify the main functions affected. Because paradoxical vocal fold movement also co-occurs with cough it can be typical to ask questions about possible paradoxical vocal fold movement symptoms during the case history interview. It is helpful to determine which symptoms are most problematic for the patient. Some patients may have equally severe cough and dysphonia, but only be concerned about one of those issues. The case history interview helps to establish rapport with the patient and offers the speech pathologist an opportunity to appreciate the patient's understanding of their symptoms and the rationale for referral to speech pathology.

The patient's degree of concern about their cough and dyspnea needs to be ascertained and may have implications for their motivation and adherence to in therapy. It may influence the degree of education and psychosocial support required throughout the treatment program. At one end of the spectrum, patients may be extremely concerned and frustrated by their cough, experience a significant impact on their daily life and feel helpless at the inability of medical treatments to relieve their symptoms. Other patients may seek help due to pressure from family members but be relatively unconcerned about their symptoms.

Patients may raise unexpected concerns, such as the cough being a sign of serious medical disease, or that a significant finding has been overlooked during their medical assessment. Others may express frustration about the cough interfering with their interpersonal relationships.

Similar to the case history used in the assessment of voice disorders, it is important to ascertain information regarding the onset, duration and progression of the cough and paradoxical vocal fold movement symptoms. Some patients have had symptoms for many years and find it difficult to recall details surrounding onset. Others will be able to recall the specific details surrounding onset of their condition. For many, the onset occurs following an upper respiratory tract infection where cough symptoms persist well after resolution of the initial infection. Other patients may report that the onset occurred after a stressful event or other serious medical illness.

Cough symptoms

The next set of questions in the case history interview relates to specific cough characteristics including cough triggers, the urge to cough, presence of deliberate coughing, cough description, cough pattern and strategies used to control the cough. Information relating to these specific characteristics of the cough can be useful in tailoring treatment programs to individual patients and is described in more detail in Chapter 10.[7]

Cough triggers

Triggers for the cough can be identified through open ended questioning or through responses to questions about specific triggers. Some patients can easily identify their cough triggers with open ended questions such as *"What triggers your cough?"* Other patients may be unable to recall information about triggers, but can identify specific triggers when asked targeted questions. The case history form [Appendix 1] includes information about the specific triggers commonly associated with chronic refractory cough. Each trigger is rated as either *present*, *absent*, or *not applicable*. The rating of *not applicable* means that the individual is not exposed to the particular trigger. This rating enables differentiation between patients who are exposed to a particular trigger which does not cause cough, and patients who are not exposed to that particular trigger. Some patients are unable to identify a particular pattern of triggers, which often causes them frustration. Reassurance may be needed that the cough may be due to general hypersensitivity and that identifying triggers is not essential for treatment to progress. Talking and laughing are significant cough triggers for many patients,[8] which suggests that vocal fold movement during phonation might stimulate cough receptors. As discussed in Chapter 6, abnormal laryngeal sensation is almost universally reported in patients with chronic refractory cough, and acts as a cough trigger.

Urge to cough and warning before cough

As described in Chapter 2, the sense of the urge to cough occurs before the actual cough behaviour. For some patients, the urge to cough is more problematic for them than the actual cough. The strength of the urge to cough can be estimated reliably using the Urge to Cough Scale developed by Davenport[9] as shown in Table 2.1. Patients can also describe the urge to cough sensation, for example a tickle or an itch. Some patients do not experience any throat sensation before coughing.[7] These individuals may have reduced awareness of their laryngeal sensation, which may need to be addressed in therapy.

Deliberate coughing

It is useful to determine whether or not the patient coughs deliberately. Most patients with chronic refractory cough have an increased sensation of laryngeal irritation.[8] Approximately 25% to 33% of patients with chronic refractory cough report that they cough deliberately in response to an uncomfortable sensation in their throat.[7] For some, it is due to a sensation of phlegm in the throat, while for others it is uncomfortable throat irritation. In these cases it would appear that the urge to cough is the primary distressing complaint and that deliberate coughing is used to relieve the urge.

Cough description

The cough may be moist or dry and may be initiated from the chest or throat. The majority of patients with chronic refractory cough have a dry irritated cough that is initiated in the throat. This differs from the pattern of infectious cough that is moist and often triggered in the chest. Identifying the throat as the source of the cough can be helpful for the patient to understand the role of the larynx in their cough. The patient may indicate that the cough is initiated from both the chest and throat, whereas some are unaware of where the cough is initiated. Some patients report that they have been complaining about their throat for years but that medical investigations have focused on the chest. The pattern of cough is also interesting. The majority of patients report that cough occurs in bouts with symptom free periods, while a smaller proportion will complain of continual coughing throughout the day.

Strategies used to control the cough

Patients may have used various strategies to control their cough. The type and effectiveness of those strategies may provide insight into how much control patients are attempting to exert over their cough and the extent to which they have internalised locus of control over their cough. Some patients will report using no strategies, while others may have tried a range of pharmaceutical or other alternatives. The majority of patients report that their strategies have been ineffective in controlling their cough. A small percentage of patients report that they drink water in attempt to control their cough and that it is ineffective. This does not, however, negate the need for adequate hydration and incorporation of water into treatment protocols.

Sensation after cough

The sensation experienced by the patient after coughing correlates to the final stage in the Urge to Cough Model, described in Chapter 2, i.e. the reward from cough. The patient may feel relieved after coughing, which might indicate that they perceive cough as a positive phenomenon. These patients may be getting positive reinforcement from their cough and may be reluctant to voluntarily suppress their cough during therapy. Other patients may have negative connotations associated with their cough, for example feeling exhausted.

Paradoxical vocal fold movement symptoms

The aim of questioning about paradoxical vocal fold movement symptoms is to determine whether or not they are present and if so, to differentiate them from other respiratory disorders such as dysfunctional breathing and asthma. Some patients may have undiagnosed paradoxical vocal fold movement in combination with their cough. Patients with combined cough and paradoxical vocal fold movement may find it difficult to differentiate between cough and paradoxical vocal fold movement symptoms, particularly if the cough occurs in conjunction with episodes of dyspnea. Some patients may primarily complain of paradoxical vocal fold movement, but on specific questioning, have significantly increased cough symptoms. The cough may occur in attempt to release glottal constriction during an episode of paradoxical vocal fold movement.[31]

Patients with paradoxical vocal fold movement are more likely to report associated throat tightness, more difficulty with inspiration than expiration, and that dyspnoeic episodes usually have a rapid onset and resolution. Triggers to the breathing symptoms typically include exercise, heart burn, post nasal drip, pollution, cold air and talking. Asthma medications rarely give relief. There can be associated dysphonia, a sensation of a lump in the throat, choking and suffocation. For some, the paradoxical vocal fold movement episodes are inextricably linked with cough episodes. Some patients report extremely severe episodes where they perceive they are going to pass out, suffocate, choke or die. Although the assessment may differentiate between paradoxical vocal fold movement and asthma symptoms, it is beyond the role of speech pathologist to diagnose or treat asthma.

Inspiration versus expiration

Difficulty with inspiration is characteristic of paradoxical vocal fold movement whereas difficulty with expiration is more characteristic of asthma. Therefore it is important to ask patients whether inspiration is more difficult than expiration. Some patients are easily able to identify whether inspiration or expiration is affected while others are unable to detect a difference.

Throat and chest tightness

Throat tightness is a characteristic symptom in of paradoxical vocal fold movement. In contrast, chest tightness is more consistent with asthma. Patients usually point to the laryngeal area when asked to locate the source of the breathing obstruction.

Inspiratory stridor

Inspiratory stridor is a characteristic feature of paradoxical vocal fold movement. Stridor is distinct from wheeze that occurs during expiration. Stridor may be present consistently or only during deep inhalation. Many patients are unfamiliar with the term *stridor* and may refer to this noise as a *wheeze*. Some patients may be able to demonstrate or mimic the noise that they make. If the patient is unable to mimic their stridor, the speech pathologist can demonstrate stridor and ask the patient or relative whether the noise they make is character-istic of this demonstration.

Sensation of suffocation

A sensation of suffocation, strangulation, and choking are often reported by patients with paradoxical vocal fold movement. Patients may report a sensation of air hunger where they perceive they are unable to inspire sufficient air. This sensation may be present in patients who initially deny inspiratory dyspnea.

Effectiveness of inhaled bronchodilators

Bronchodilators are used in the treatment of asthma and are known as asthma relievers. Patients with paradoxical vocal fold movement may report that bron-chodilators are ineffective in relieving their respiratory symptoms, or that relief is not achieved without excessive doses of the medication. Patients with con-firmed asthma may have paradoxical vocal fold movement that presents as a worsening, or change in asthma symptoms. Many patients with co-existing asthma may have taken escalating doses of various asthma medications without substantial benefit.[10]

Onset and resolution of dyspnea episodes

The length of time it takes for symptoms to emerge in response to a stimulus, and to resolve once the triggering stimulus has been removed, should be clari-fied. Patients with paradoxical vocal fold movement typically report that the onset of episodes occurs within less than five minutes of exposure to a particular trigger. In contrast, onset of symptoms lasting longer than five minutes is less characteristic of paradoxical vocal fold movement and may be more consistent with asthma. Resolution of symptoms within five minutes is characteristic of paradoxical vocal fold movement whereas longer than five minutes is more sug-gestive of asthma.

Medical history

The medical history is a critical component of the speech pathology assessment. In some cases, a thorough medical history will have been provided by the refer-ring doctor and may simply require clarification during the case history inter-view. The speech pathologist should note the presence of diseases frequently associated with chronic refractory cough and paradoxical vocal fold movement, including gastroesophageal reflux disease, rhinosinusitis, Angiotensin Convert-ing Enzyme (ACE) inhibitor use, asthma, and obstructive sleep apnoea. The majority of these issues will have been investigated prior to referral to speech pathology. Other medical conditions, previous surgery or traumatic injuries, medications, treatments, and social history should also be noted. Current or previous medical treatment for the medical conditions associated with chronic refractory cough should also be noted. In many cases, medical treatment might be effective for the underlying condition but have no effect on the cough. For example, medical treatment for cough associated with gastroesophageal reflux disease might reduce reflux symptoms such as heartburn, but have no effect on the severity or frequency of cough.

Gastroesophageal and laryngopharyngeal reflux

Typical reflux symptoms may include heartburn and indigestion, although many patients with reflux may be asymptomatic. Specific information regarding previ-ous and current anti-reflux treatment should be ascertained. This information includes the presence and type of reflux treatment, including pharmaceutical and lifestyle modifications. Patient compliance with reflux treatment should also be determined. Some patients may give up on a trial of proton pump inhibi-tors early if they do not see immediate improvement in their symptoms. Others may have been given lifestyle modifications by their treating doctor but not implemented them. Further education may be required to facilitate the patient's understanding of the rationale for these recommendations. Finally, the effec-tiveness of reflux treatment on both the underlying condition, i.e. the reflux symptoms, and on the cough should be noted. Reflux treatment may have a pos-itive effect on the underlying reflux symptoms but have no effect on the cough. If reflux treatment improves reflux symptoms but not the cough, it suggests that either the cough is not due to reflux or that the patient has non-acidic reflux.

Asthma

It is important to know whether or not the patient has asthma, and if so, how asthma was diagnosed, when it was last reviewed, current medications, cur-rent asthma management plan and inhaler technique. Some patients may have been given an asthma diagnosis many years previously based on symptoms and response to bronchodilators but without a comprehensive diagnostic assessment. Such patients continue to carry the *asthma* label when they may not in fact have asthma. A formal asthma review may be required if it has not occurred in the last two years and the patient's symptoms are suggestive of asthma. The speech pathologist should determine whether asthma treatment has been effective in both controlling the asthma symptoms and controlling the cough. If ineffective in controlling the asthma, it might suggest unstable asthma that requires review. Alternatively, asthma medication may be effective for asthma symptoms such as shortness of breath and wheeze, but have no effect on the underlying cough. This phenomenon would suggest that cough is not due to asthma.

Paradoxical vocal fold movement can co-occur with asthma. Paradoxical vocal fold movement might initially present as a worsening of asthma symptoms. Asthma medication is ineffective in treating paradoxical vocal fold movement episodes. Some patients can easily distinguish between the asthma and paradoxical vocal fold movement exacerbations whereas others have more difficulty.

Rhinosinusitis

Patients with rhinosinusitis may have rhinitis, post nasal drip or sinus disease. The significance of these symptoms is difficult to judge as some patients have heightened sensation to normally occurring mucous production. Similar to asthma and reflux it is important to determine whether any previous medical treatment of rhinitis has been effective in relieving both the rhinitis symptoms and the cough.

Obstructive sleep apnoea

Obstructive sleep apnoea can be associated with chronic refractory cough and may be diagnosed through a sleep study. Obstructive sleep apnoea has been less routinely examined in patients with cough. It may be suggested if patients or their partners report cessation of breathing during the night or daytime somnolence. Specific screening questionnaires for obstructive sleep apnoea are available.

ACE Inhibitors

It is important to note whether or not a trial of withdrawing ACE inhibitor medication has occurred and whether or not it has been effective in reducing cough. A trial may need to be considered even if there is no temporal association between commencing ACE inhibitors and onset of the cough.

Results of diagnostic testing

In addition to understanding the medical history and effects of previous medical treatment for cough, the speech pathologist should understand the results of medical investigations that have been conducted. As stated in Chapters 3, 4, and 5, typical investigations used in the assessment of the patient with chronic refractory cough include nasendoscopy, pulmonary function testing, challenge testing, chest radiographs, and bronchoscopy.

Pulmonary function testing

Pulmonary function testing, cough reflex sensitivity testing (see Appendix 7) and hypertonic saline challenge are described in Chapter 4. These tests are generally administered by respiratory technicians, however speech pathologists can be trained to perform the tests in some settings. The results of pulmonary function testing form a useful part of the patient profile. Although it is not the role of the speech pathologist to diagnose respiratory disease, pulmonary function test results can help the speech pathologist to form a more holistic view of the patient's condition. It can be reassuring to know whether or not baseline pulmonary function test results are within the normal range, particularly in patients complaining of respiratory symptoms. The results of challenge testing may suggest asthma or paradoxical vocal fold movement. For example, a fall in FIF_{50} after provocation with hypertonic saline challenge of more than 20% may be suggestive of paradoxical vocal fold movement. In contrast, a fall in FEV_1 of more than 15% is suggestive of asthma. A fall in FEV_1 of less than 15% suggests that either the individual does not have asthma, or that their asthma is well controlled.

Chest radiograph

Most patients with chronic refractory cough will have had a chest radiograph performed by their primary care physician prior to referral to a respiratory physician or speech pathologist. Chest radiographs are used in chronic refractory cough to exclude pathology such as pulmonary malignancy, cardiac failure, interstitial lung disease, bronchiectasis, or tuberculosis, that may also cause cough.[11] Chest radiographs are usually normal in patients referred to specialist cough clinics,[12] and patients with abnormal findings are rarely referred to speech pathology for management of their cough. They may be also used in the differential diagnosis of paradoxical vocal fold movement to eliminate pulmonary causes of the dyspnea.

Bronchoscopy

There is variation in clinical practice regarding referring patients with chronic refractory cough for bronchoscopy. Bronchoscopy is generally performed if the clinician suspects underlying pathology. Results are frequently normal in patients referred to speech pathology for chronic refractory cough

Hydration and vocally traumatic behaviours

Many patients with chronic refractory cough have poor vocal hygiene, which may exacerbate laryngeal irritation. Assessment of vocal hygiene is familiar to most speech pathologists. Phonotraumatic vocal behaviours include shouting, loud talking, screaming, vocal noises, coughing, throat clearing, and extensive voice use. The effect of behaviours, such as loud or extensive talking, will vary between patients and, in fact, may not be detrimental for some individuals. For example, loud talking may not be detrimental if there is adequate respiratory support and oral resonance, and the individual is well hydrated.

Hydration and laryngeal irritation are also examined. These factors include water intake, and other factors known to exacerbate irritation such as smoking, alcohol, drugs, caffeine, oral rather than nasal breathing, cough lozenges, poor sleep, and exposure to fumes. The exact quantity of alcohol, water and caffeine consumed is preferable to general descriptions such as *"not much"* or *"a lot"*, which can be inaccurate or open to interpretation.

Symptom ratings and questionnaires

The next component of the speech pathology assessment of the patient with chronic refractory cough involves symptom ratings. Symptom ratings provide a cost effective and non-invasive method of quantifying symptoms from the patient's perspective, and understanding the patient's particular symptom profile. These ratings can indicate the severity of the problem, provide baseline data, and be used to measure change following treatment. Various tools are available which measure different aspects of impairment, and commonly used scales are reported in the following sections. The choice of rating scale will depend upon the patient's clinical presentation.

Symptom frequency and severity scale

The John Hunter Hospital Symptom Frequency and Severity scale (Appendix 2) can be used to measure a range of voice, upper airway, respiratory and cough symptoms. This scale includes the rating of the frequency, severity and limitation of various cough, respiratory, voice and upper airway symptoms. The frequencies of 19 different symptoms are each rated on a five-point scale from 1 (*never present*) to 5 (*present all the time*). The severity of breathing, cough, voice and upper airway symptoms is rated on a five-point scale from 1 (*absent, none at all*) to 5 (*most severe discomfort ever*). Finally, the limitation of symptoms on day-to-day activity is rated on a five-point scale from 1 (*not limited, have done all the activities that I want to*) to 5 (*severely limited*). Patients circle the number that corresponds to the rating in each question. Five subscale scores are calculated from the symptom rating data and include a total symptom score, breathing score, cough score, voice score and upper airway score. The total symptom score is calculated by adding all the frequency (19), severity (4) and limitation (1) scores, and subtracting 24 to adjust for the normal rating being given a score of 1. The breathing score is calculated by adding the five frequency and severity scores pertaining to breathing, and subtracting 5. The cough score is calculated by adding the four frequency and severity scores pertaining to cough, and subtracting 4. The voice score is calculated by adding the six frequency and severity scores pertaining to voice, and subtracting 6. The upper airway score is calculated by adding the seven frequency and severity scores pertaining to upper airway symptoms, and subtracting 7. These scores can be obtained by inputting the numbers into the Author's symptom frequency and severity rating Excel spreadsheet available through the Publisher. This spreadsheet calculates the composite scores for each patient and provides normative data. Normal symptom frequency and severity scores are outlined in Table 8.2. These scores have proved to be significantly different between healthy controls and individuals with chronic refractory cough or paradoxical vocal fold movement and to demonstrate significant improvement following successful treatment.

Composite score	Norm
Total symptom score	< 15.4
Breathing score	< 4.1
Cough score	< 6.2
Voice score	< 5.7
Upper airway score	< 5.8

Table 8.2: John Hunter Hospital Symptom Frequency and Severity Scale norms

125

Leicester Cough Questionnaire

Cough quality of life questionnaires are useful to measure the psychosocial impacts of cough, and are useful outcome measures. The Leicester Cough Questionnaire (LCQ)[13] (Appendix 3) is a self-administered questionnaire about various symptoms pertaining to cough quality of life, in which patients rate 19 items on a seven-point Likert scale, ranging from 1 (*all of the time*) to 7 (*none of the time*). Items are attributed to either of physical, social or psychological domains. The physical domain includes items 1, 2, 3, 9, 10, 11, 14, and 15; the social domain includes items 7, 8, 18, and 19; and the psychological domain includes items 4, 5, 6, 12, 13, 16, and 17. Domain scores are calculated by dividing the total score from items in the domain and dividing by the number of items in the domain. The range of possible domain scores is between 1 and 7. The total score is the addition of domain scores. The range of possible total scores is between 3 and 21.

Reflux Symptom Index

The Reflux Symptom Index,[14] is a reliable and valid self-report measure of the severity of laryngopharyngeal reflux symptoms. It documents the presence and severity of nine symptoms of laryngopharyngeal reflux. This scale does not diagnose reflux, but measures the severity of symptoms relating to laryngopharyngeal reflux. Symptoms are rated on a five point scale, with scores 13 or above considered abnormal. The Reflux Symptom Index can provide useful information regarding symptoms of laryngopharyngeal reflux.[14] This index monitors change in symptoms of laryngopharyngeal reflux following medical treatment.

Voice Handicap Index

Voice symptoms can occur in patients with chronic refractory cough. The Voice Handicap Index[15] is an easy method for documenting the severity of voice-related quality of life and is routinely used in the management of voice disorders. The Voice Handicap Index contains 30 items, rated on a 5 point scale from 0 (*never*) to 4 (*always*). There are three subscale scores: physical, emotional and functional. Total scores of 0 to 19 are considered normal; 20 to 39, mild; 41 to 59, moderate; and 60 and above, severe.

Newcastle Laryngeal Hypersensitivity Questionnaire

The Newcastle Laryngeal Hypersensitivity Questionnaire[16] is a valid measure of laryngeal discomfort for patients with laryngeal hypersensitivity syndromes. It contains 14 items with a 7 point Likert frequency response scale (see Appendix 4). It is designed for self-administration and takes less than 5 minutes for completion. The questionnaire is useful in discriminating between patients with laryngeal hypersensitivity syndromes and healthy controls, and is able to detect a change in laryngeal hypersensitivity after speech pathology treatment. The cut-off for normal function is 17.1. Questionnaire scoring is in a similar direction to the Leicester Cough Questionnaire. Subscale scores are averaged from the number of completed items for each subscale and range from 1 (*worst*) to 7 (*best*). The total score is the sum of the three subscale scores, which range from 3 (*worst*) to 21 (*best*). The minimal important difference is 1.7. The Laryngeal Hypersensitivity Questionnaire has a number of purposes, including quantifying the patient experience of laryngeal discomfort, and measuring change over time and outcome of treatment. It can discriminate between patient groups and healthy controls.

Dyspnea Index

The Dyspnea Index[17] is a 10-item questionnaire of symptoms related to respiratory difficulty. Items are rated on a five-point scale ranging from 0 (*almost never*) to 4 (*always*). Scores above 10 are in the abnormal range. The Dyspnea Index evaluates overall symptom severity of dyspnea in patients with a range of upper airway pathologies, and is a useful outcome measure.

Cough Severity Index

The Cough Severity Index[18] is similar to the Dyspnea Index and contains 10 items related to cough symptoms. Items are rated on a five-point scale ranging from 0 (almost never) to 4 (always). Scores above 3.23 (i.e. the mean, plus two standard deviations for healthy controls) are considered abnormal. The Cough Severity Index is not used for diagnosis of cough, but to quantify the patient perception of cough. It has strong test-retest reliability and discriminant validity to differentiate patients from healthy controls. Scores also show significant reduction following successful behavioural treatment of cough.

Clinical observations and non-instrumental assessment

Following the case history and symptom ratings, a number of clinical observations and tests should be utilised. These tests are easy to administer and will be familiar to speech pathologists who manage patients with voice disorders. This component of the assessment does not require instrumentation. Details are outlined below and summarised in Appendix 5.

Oromusculature/cranial nerve assessment

In the vast majority of cases, the oromusculature/cranial nerve examination is normal. However, with the emergence of literature regarding sensory neuropathy and cough, it could be prudent to conduct a brief screening of cranial nerve function. Cranial nerve assessment is familiar to speech pathologists. The oromusculature assessment may reveal the presence of a dry mouth or hypersensitive gag reflex.

Swallowing

Oropharyngeal dysphagia is not suspected in the majority of patients with chronic refractory cough. However, many patients with chronic refractory cough report globus type symptoms and on specific questioning, may describe swallowing symptoms. A brief swallowing assessment may detect the possibility of oropharyngeal dysphagia, which requires more comprehensive investigation, particularly if aspiration is suspected as a cause of cough. This assessment can involve assessment of reflexive swallow while sipping water and during continuous drinking, observations of oral control and palpation of hyolaryngeal excursion and cervical auscultation. The Timed Swallow Test[19] is useful for quantifying swallowing efficiency. Interestingly, although patients with chronic refractory cough have Timed Swallow Test values within the normal range, they are reduced when compared to healthy controls.[20] The underlying mechanism for these results is unclear.

Respiration

A number of observations should be made regarding respiration including the habitual pattern of breathing, breathing difficulty, stridor, and breath holding. The patient's habitual pattern of breathing should be noted, particularly the presence of shallow breathing or excess shoulder movement during respiration.[21] The breathing pattern is classified as clavicular, thoracic, diaphragmatic, or abdominal. The breathing route is classified as oral, nasal, or combined. Breathing difficulty may include mouth breathing, struggling for air, gasping, or effortful inhalation. Inspiratory stridor may be present and is a sign of paradoxical vocal fold movement. Stridor may be present at rest, or may only be present during deep inspiration or physical exertion. The degree of breath-holding should be determined including whether it is present and the conditions under which it occurs. For example, does breath-holding occur frequently during the case history interview, or after a specified precipitant (such as when attempting to suppress cough), during concentration, or movement? Some patients hold their breath unconsciously. This habit may increase the sensation of breathlessness and contribute to increased laryngeal constriction. Simply bringing the patient's attention to their breath-holding may be sufficient to address this behaviour. Respiratory rate should be measured.

The coordination of respiration and phonation during connected speech, such as monologue or reading, may reveal difficulty that is not evident during conversation. During general conversation, the length of utterance, pausing and phrasing should be observed. Observation of respiration during formal voice assessment tasks, such as vowel prolongation, pitch glides and tests of vocal fatigue, will provide useful information about respiratory control and respiration.

Posture and tension

Excess neck and shoulder tension may be observed at rest, during conversational speech or during specific exercises. Stemple[21] reports increased muscle tension in 75% of patients with irritable larynx syndrome, and suggests observing the patient to determine whether tension is held in back or abdominal muscles. Tension may be more prevalent when the patient performs a physical activity such as walking, moving from sitting to standing, or picking up an object from the floor. Extrinsic laryngeal muscle tension may be felt by palpating the extrinsic laryngeal musculature, namely the thyrohyoid and genio hyoid regions. Murry[22] recommends laryngeal palpation of the suprahyoid and infrahyoid muscles at rest, during inspiration and expiration and during the initiation of phonation. The shoulders and chest should also be observed during phonation and quiet breathing. Stemple[21] suggests observing for eyebrow adduction, clenched jaw, scalloped tongue, and tension between the maxilla and mandible.

Cough

Observations of cough and throat clearing should be made during the assessment. These observations include a description of the type and pattern of the cough, and identifiable triggers. Throat clearing should be distinguished from cough. This is characterised by glottal adduction and forced expiration without the preceding inspiratory phase seen in cough.

The patient's attempts to suppress their cough, and the degree to which they are aware of coughing and throat clearing are also important to record. In many cases, however, individuals with chronic refractory cough might not cough during the assessment and therefore, the speech pathologist might not have the opportunity to observe the patient's cough behaviour.

Voice screening

Approximately 40% of patients with chronic refractory cough and paradoxical vocal fold movement have clinically significant voice disorders.[23] Therefore, as a minimum it is recommended that voice screening be conducted in the assessment of chronic refractory cough. While voice problems can be significant in chronic refractory cough, patients may be primarily concerned about their cough and relatively unconcerned about their voice.

Formal voice assessment tasks, such as vowel prolongation, scales and glides can trigger cough, even if cough is not observed during other parts of the assessment. Furthermore, these tasks can increase the patient's urge to cough even if they do not trigger a cough;[20] perhaps because these tasks extend the voice to the limits of pitch, loudness and duration. Further objective studies with controlled vocal loading are required to measure the effect of phonation as a cough trigger.

Non-instrumental voice assessment tasks can easily be included in the initial assessment protocol and provide information on vocal fatigue, prolongation times, pitch and loudness. More comprehensive assessment of vocal function including instrumental measures should be conducted in individuals who report voice changes or problems, those who present with disordered voice quality during the case history interview, those with a concern about their voice, severe dysphonia, and professional voice users. Measures of vocal function can serve as additional outcome measures for patients presenting with coexisting voice problems.

The voice screening protocol is incorporated into Appendix 5 and includes (1) auditory perceptual evaluation of vocal quality, pitch, loudness, and resonance during conversation and reading; (2) maximum phonation time; (3) pitch range, e.g. perceptual judgement of pitch ranges during scale and glide tasks; (4) loudness range, e.g. perceptual judgement of loudness during habitual speaking and phonation at the patient's minimum and maximum volume; (5) laryngeal diadachokinesis, i.e. rapid glottal attacks; (6) test for vocal fatigue, e.g. judging deterioration in voice or cough while counting from 1 to 50; (7) coordination of respiration and phonation; (8) soft high pitched phonation on sustained /i/, repetition of /hi/, soft ascending pitch glide, and high soft singing; and (9) observation of phonotraumatic vocal behaviours. Phonotraumatic vocal behaviours may be present, and may contribute to cough and laryngeal irritation. These behaviours include throat clearing, hard glottal attacks, laryngeal focus of resonance, reduced breath support, throat clearing to initiate phonation, and inappropriate pitch or loudness. The presence of these behaviours during the assessment and the extent to which they contribute to cough should be noted.

Voice Stress Test

The Voice Stress Test has been adapted by Awan[26] and may result in a deterioration of voice quality, increased urge to cough and increased cough frequency.[20]

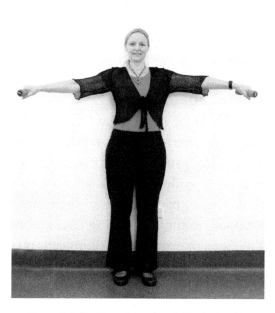

Figure 8.1: Position of hand weights during the Voice Stress Test

The Voice Stress Test starts with baseline measures of urge to cough and vocal quality. The patient then holds one kilogram hand weights extended in a lateral position as shown in Figure 8.1. This lateral position is held for one minute, and during this time, the patient reads the second line of the Rainbow Passage.[27] *"The rainbow is a division of white light into many beautiful colours,"* and then prolongs the phoneme /a/ for as long as possible. This sequence is repeated several times for one minute. The urge-to-cough, vocal quality, and cough count are measured during the following 30 seconds. The phonation sequence, followed by the urge to cough, voice quality and cough count measures, are then repeated for a second time.

Urge to Cough and triggers assessment

In addition to patient self-report of cough triggers, formal exposure to potential triggers can be trialled in the clinical setting.[22] This assessment is shown in Appendix 6. In this assessment, both the magnitude of the Urge to Cough[9] and the number of coughs observed are rated at baseline and then after exposure to various olfactory, exercise, phonatory, respiratory, and swallowing triggers. These triggers include deep inspiration, reading aloud, exercise, voice assessment tasks, perfume, soap powder, eating, and drinking. In addition to judging urge to cough after exposure to potentially triggering stimuli, patients can also be coached in strategies to relieve the urge to cough. This assessment process can raise the patient's awareness of the transience of the urge to cough, and the potential for it to be modified through environmental changes.

Psychological screening

Although psychiatric and psychological issues cannot automatically be assumed in patients with chronic refractory cough and paradoxical vocal fold movement, there is potential for these factors to occur in individual cases. It may be helpful to ascertain the patient's perception of whether or not symptoms fluctuate according to stress. This reflection provides an opportunity for patients to reflect upon stress and emotion as potentially predisposing, or exacerbating factors in their condition. It invites the patient to evaluate the role of stress in their condition, rather than suggest that stress may be the cause of symptoms.

Psychological screening tests such as the Hospital Anxiety and Depression Scale[24] can be useful to indicate an individual's current anxiety and depression status. Psychological screening tests can be readministered at the conclusion of intervention, to monitor change in psychological symptoms. It is advisable for speech pathologists to consult with psychologists or psychiatrists in their mental health teams for further training and support in these screening tests and to avoid diagnosing or working outside of their area of expertise. A significant rating on a psychological screening test, or significant psychological issues arising from the case history should promote discussion of the possibility of referral to a mental health professional.

If psychological symptoms improve following resolution of the cough, then anxiety and depression issues could be assumed to be a result rather than a cause of the cough. However, it is difficult to discount the non-specific therapeutic benefits of speech pathology intervention, such as empathy and warmth. In some cases, having someone understand their problem can be therapeutic.[25]

Diagnostic therapy

A trial of therapy should be included as part of the initial consultation.[28] This trial provides the patient with some active strategies to exert control over their cough. It also enables the speech pathologist to judge the patient's capacity to learn the exercises, which might provide some prognostic information.

Instrumental assessment

Instrumental testing may have been conducted prior to referral to speech pathology, or might be conducted as part of the speech pathology assessment. This testing may include nasendoscopy, laryngeal videostroboscopy, pulmonary function testing, cough reflex sensitivity testing, instrumental voice assessment, ambulatory cough monitoring, and hypertonic saline challenge. Some patients primarily complain of cough, but are found to have paradoxical vocal fold movement on instrumental testing.

Nasendoscopy

Nasendoscopy can be helpful in determining the presence or absence of laryngeal lesions, signs of laryngopharyngeal reflux, and abnormal laryngeal movements during respiration and phonation. Nasendoscopy can also help diagnose paradoxical vocal fold movement, although it may also result in false negatives if the procedure is conducted while the patient is asymptomatic. Ideally, nasendoscopy should be performed with some sort of provocation, such as exercise or an inhaled irritant.

Nasendoscopy may have been performed prior to referral to speech pathology, or might be performed as part of the speech pathology assessment. Alternatively, the speech pathologist might refer the patient for nasendoscopy assessment. It should be noted that signs of paradoxical vocal fold movement may not be evident if conducted while the patient is asymptomatic.

The nasendoscopy assessment protocol reported by Forrest[29] examines the larynx during provocation. The larynx is observed at rest. There may be twitching of the arytenoid cartilages.[21] The patient is instructed to breathe in and out through the nose, then in through the nose and out through the mouth, and finally in and out through the mouth. They then hold their breath for five seconds and release, count from one to ten on one breath, and then count for as long as possible on one breath. Although not part of the Forrest protocol, we have included vocalization tasks such as sustained vowels, pitch and loudness range tasks and connected speech samples. If paradoxical vocal fold movement is noted during any of these manoeuvres, the speech pathologist will coach the patient in breathing exercises to relieve the symptoms.

Following these tasks, the patient is exposed to an odour challenge. We use cheap perfume sprayed onto cotton wool inside a cup. If the perfume challenge triggers paradoxical vocal fold movement, the speech pathologist will coach the patient in the breathing exercises. If no paradoxical vocal fold movement is observed, the scope is removed and patients are coached in exertion, such as climbing stairs or riding an exercise bike. The scope is reinserted to observe for any signs of paradoxical vocal fold movement.

Instrumental voice assessment

Instrumental voice assessment including acoustic, aerodynamic and electroglottographic measures may be appropriate for some patients, particularly if significant dysphonia is identified during screening. It is assumed that speech pathologists are familiar with these instrumental voice assessments.

Ambulatory cough monitoring

Ambulatory cough monitoring provides objective information about the frequency and timing of cough episodes. The Leicester Cough Monitor, shown in Figure 8.2, is a small recording device which is worn around the neck for 24 hours. It records all coughing and clearing behaviours. The recordings are downloaded to a computer program for analysis.

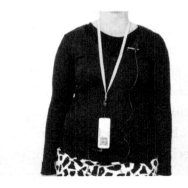

Figure 8.2: Leicester Cough Monitor.

Diagnosis

Once the assessment is completed, the speech pathologist will determine the severity of the problem and summarise the etiological and maintaining factors, including associated medical conditions. The speech pathologist can diagnose the patient as having a laryngeal sensory hyperresponsiveness syndrome, or alternatively, might make a more specific diagnosis such as:

1. Paradoxical Vocal Fold Movement.
2. Chronic refractory cough.
3. Exercise induced paradoxical vocal fold movement.
4. Irritant induced paradoxical vocal fold movement.
5. Combined paradoxical vocal fold movement and asthma.
6. Muscle Tension Dysphonia.
7. Globus pharyngeus.
8. Dysfunctional breathing.

The management of these conditions will differ, although there may be some overlap in the approach and goals of therapy, such as improving voluntary control over symptoms and reducing laryngeal irritation. Although the patient may be referred to the speech pathologist with a diagnosis of chronic cough, the speech pathology assessment might reveal a different or coexisting condition, such as muscle tension dysphonia or globus pharyngeus. Such patients may benefit from a traditional voice therapy program for management of these coexisting conditions.[32]

The assessment might indicate that speech pathology intervention is not appropriate for that individual, or that additional diagnostic information is required before determining eligibility for the treatment. Speech pathologists should feel justified in withholding or delaying intervention in situations where it is not deemed appropriate.

Summary

The assessment of the patient with chronic refractory cough involves a detailed case history interview including description of cough, breathing and voice symptoms. Associated medication conditions have usually been addressed prior to assessment by the speech pathologist; nevertheless the clinician should be alert to the contribution of these conditions to the progression of symptoms. A range of patient rating scales are available to determine the severity at baseline, and to measure change over time. Clinical observation and non-instrumental assessment of oromusculature function, respiration, cough, and voice can be easily conducted in the clinical setting. Instrumental assessment is invaluable in identifying the underlying physiology of cough and laryngeal behaviour.

References

1. Gay M, Blager F, Bartsch K, Emery C. Psychogenic habit cough: Review and case reports. *Journal of Child Psychiatry*. 1987;48(12):483–6.

2. Gibson P, Chang A, Glasgow N, Holmes P, Katelaris P, Kemp A, *et al*. Cough In Children and Adults, Diagnosis and Assessment: Australian Cough Guidelines. *Medical Journal of Australia*. 2010;192(5):265–71.

3. Gibson PG, Wang G, McGarvey L, Vertigan A, Altman K, SS B. Treatment of Unexplained Chronic Cough: CHEST Guideline and Expert Panel Report. *Chest*. 2015;in press.

4. Vertigan A, Theodoros D, Winkworth A, Gibson P. Chronic cough: A tutorial for speech language pathologists. *Journal of Medical Speech Language Pathology*. 2007;15:189–206.

5. Barsky A, Borus J. Functional somatic syndromes. *Annals of Internal Medicine*. 1999;130:910–21.

6. Russell A. Non-medical management of chronic persistent cough. Paper presented at the *Australian Association of Speech and Hearing conference*; Adelaide, Australia, 1991.

7. Vertigan A, Theodoros D, Gibson P, Winkworth A. Voice and upper airway symptoms in people with chronic cough and paradoxical vocal fold movement. *Journal of Voice*. 2007;21(3):361–83.

8. Vertigan A, Gibson P. Chronic refractory cough as a laryngeal sensory neuropathy: Evidence from a reinterpretation of cough triggers. *Journal of Voice*. 2011;25(5):596–601.

9. Davenport P, Sapienza C, Bolser D. Psychophysical assessment of the urge to cough. *European Respiratory Journal*. 2002;12:249–53.

10. Brugman S. What's this thing called vocal cord dysfunction? *Primary and Critical Care Update*. 2006;20(26).

11. Ing A, Breslin A. The patient with chronic cough. *Medical Journal of Australia*. 1997;166:491–6.

12. McGarvey L. Cough 6: Which investigations are most useful in the diagnois of chronic cough? *Thorax*. 2004;59:342–6.

13. Birring S, Prudon B, Carr A, *et al*. Development of a symptom specific health status measure for patients with chronic cough: Leicester Cough Questionnaire. *Thorax*. 2003;58:339–43.

14. Belafsky P, Potsma G, Koufman J. Validity and reliability of the reflux symptom index (RSI). *Journal of Voice*. 2002;16(2):274–7.

15. Jacobson H, Johnson A, Grywalski C, *et al*. The voice handicap index (VHI): Development and validation. *American Journal of Speech Language Pathology*. 1997;6:66–70.

16. Vertigan AE, Bone SL, Gibson PG. Development and validation of the Newcastle laryngeal hypersensitivity questionnaire. *Cough*. 2014;10(1):1.

17. Gartner-Schmidt J, Shembel AC, Zullo T, Rosen CA. Development and validation of the dyspnea index (DI): A severity index for upper airway-related dyspnea. *Journal of Voice*. 2014;28(6):775–82.

18. Shembel AC, Rosen CA, Zullo TG, Gartner-Schmidt JL. Development and validation of the cough severity index: a severity index for chronic cough related to the upper airway. *The Laryngoscope*. 2013;123(8):1931–6.

19. Nathadwarawala K, Nicklin J, Wiles C. A timed test of swallowing capacity for neurological patients. *Journal of Neurology, Neurosurgery & Psychiatry*. 1992;55(9):822–55.

20. Vertigan A, Bone S, Gibson PG. Laryngeal sensory dysfunction in laryngeal hypersensitivity syndrome. *Respirology*. 2013;18(6):948–56.

21. Stemple J, Fry L. *Voice Therapy: Clinical Case Studies*. 3rd edn. San Diego, CA: Plural Publishing; 2009.

22. Murry T, Sapienza C. The role of voice therapy in the management of paradoxical vocal fold motion, chronic cough and laryngospasm. *Otolaryngologic Clinics of North America*. 2010;43:73–83.

23. Vertigan A, Theodoros D, Winkworth A, Gibson P. Perceptual voice characteristics in chronic cough and paradoxical vocal fold movement. *Folia Phoniatrica et Logopaedica*. 2007;59(5):256–67.

24. Zigmond A, Snaith R. The hospital anxiety and depression scale. *Acta Psychiatrica Scandinavica*. 1983;67(6):361–70.

25. Morrison M, Rammage L, Emami A. The irritable larynx syndrome. *Journal of Voice*. 1999;13(3):447–55.

26. Awan S. Effect of induced effort/strain on voice. *38th Annual Symposium: Care of the Professional Voice* 3–7 June 2009; Philadelphia, PA, USA.

27. Fairbanks G. *Voice and Articulation Drill Book* (2nd edn). New York, NY: Harper & Row; 1960.

28. Murry T, Branski R, Yu K, *et al*. Laryngeal sensory deficits in patients with chronic cough and paradoxical vocal fold movement disorder. *The Laryngoscope*. 2010;120:1576–81.

29. Forrest L, Husein T, Husein O. Paradoxical vocal cord motion: classification and treatment. *The Laryngoscope*. 2012;122:844–53.

30. Vertigan AE, Bone SL, Gibson PG. Laryngeal sensory dysfunction in laryngeal hypersensitivity syndrome. *Respirology*. 2013;18(6):948–56.

31. Blager F. Paradoxical vocal fold movement: Diagnosis and management. *Current Opinion in Otolaryngology & Head and Neck Surgery*. 2000;8:180–3.

32. Carding P, Horsley I, Docherty G. A study of the effectiveness of voice therapy in the treatment of 45 patients with nonorganic dysphonia. *Journal of Voice*. 1999;13(1):72–104.

137

Speech pathology treatment of chronic refractory cough

Anne E. Vertigan

Speech pathology treatment for chronic refractory cough follows the assessment as described in Chapter 8. This chapter outlines the treatment of patients with chronic refractory cough. It describes the John Hunter Hospital Chronic Refractory Cough (JHCRC) program, with reference to the work of other authors. A structure for developing personalised treatment plans is described in Chapter 10.

Speech pathology treatment for chronic refractory cough has two aims. The first aim is to reduce laryngeal irritation that can exacerbate cough. The second aim is to improve voluntary control over cough and respiratory symptoms, in order to teach patients to respond to the urge to cough in a manner which does not exacerbate further coughing. These two goals will ultimately reduce the frequency and severity of cough. The JHCRC speech pathology program has been developed to address these goals. It encompasses four components (1) education, (2) exercises to improve voluntary control over cough and cough suppression, (3) reduction of laryngeal irritation, including vocal hygiene training and minimising phonotrauma, and (4) psychoeducational counselling.

Education

The purpose of education is to help the patient understand the nature of chronic refractory cough and the role of behavioural therapy. This is essential to help the patient engage with the treatment program and achieve the treatment goals.

Education is provided through discussion with the patient and provision of written material. An example of the written education material is included in Appendix 8. The following issues are addressed during education:

1. **Physiology and function of the cough and larynx:** The first component of education is to provide information about the basic physiology of cough. The role of cough is to clear material from the airway. Therefore, cough has a protective function and is necessary in acute infectious cough, during aspiration or inhalation of foreign bodies. This component of the education may also include information about laryngeal anatomy and movement patterns during normal laryngeal functions, such as respiration, phonation, cough and swallowing.

2. **Abnormal laryngeal movement:** The second component includes information about abnormal movement patterns during excessive cough, throat clearing and paradoxical vocal fold movement.

3. **Side-effects of cough:** There are negative side-effects of repeated coughing, including laryngeal trauma, exacerbation of irritation, perpetuation of cough cycle. Furthermore, repeated cough increases irritation, leading to a cycle whereby irritation triggers cough which exacerbates irritation and causes further coughing. Many patients believe it is harmful to suppress a cough, particularly those who cough repeatedly in attempt to clear small amounts of phlegm. In fact, it could be the physical act of coughing that produces the small amounts of phlegm. In the majority of cases, infectious cough has been excluded by the respiratory physician prior to referral to speech pathology and it is safe to suppress the cough.

4. **Cough is not always necessary:** Although cough has a protective function it is not always necessary. In chronic refractory cough, there is a lack of physiological benefit from cough. There is nothing in the airways that requires expectoration. The patient may need to acknowledge that there is no need to cough for the reasons they think they need to cough. For example, mucous is healthy and needs to be there.[1] Patients may have hypersensitivity of the larynx and reduced thresholds for normally occurring protective behaviours.[2]

5. **Voluntary control of cough:** Many patients believe that cough is purely reflexive and that it is not possible to exert any voluntary control over their cough. However several studies have demonstrated a degree of

cortical control over cough[3] and the urge to cough is perceived by the patient before the actual cough event.[4] Patients need to understand that they can bring laryngeal behaviour under volitional control and that, as they begin to interrupt and prevent the cough, the cough will become less severe, less frequent and shorter.[1,2]

6. **Identifying the cause of the cough is not essential:** Some patients are reluctant to engage in behavioural treatment for their cough if the cause of their cough has not been determined, or if the cough persists despite treatment for that identified cause. It is helpful to reinforce that cough persists despite medical treatment in approximately 20% of patients with chronic refractory cough.

7. **The larynx may be the source of the cough and respiratory issues:** Finally, it may be necessary to increase awareness that the larynx is the source of the respiratory problem.[2]

Symptom control exercises

Cough control exercises include breathing retraining, cough control breathing, cough suppression swallow, relaxed throat breathing, distraction techniques, laryngeal deconstriction, and paradoxical vocal fold movement release breathing. The aim of cough control exercises is to prevent or interrupt cough episodes. Patients are taught to identify the precipitating sensation, warning sign, or urge to cough and then substitute the cough with a cough control technique. In other words, the cough control techniques are substituted as a competing response to cough. While the individual might experience an urge to cough, they will respond to the urge without inducing further phonotrauma.

Cough control techniques are taught in a treatment hierarchy. The techniques are initially taught in the clinical situation in the absence of any cough triggers. The aim of this first stage is for the speech pathologist to ensure that the patient is performing the exercise with the correct technique. Although at first glance, many of the techniques appear quite simple, careful attention must be paid to the patient's technique when performing the exercises. Techniques should be performed without excess laryngeal or clavicular tension, and should ensure that excess effort is not applied to the inspiratory phase of respiration.

The second stage in the treatment hierarchy involves practicing the exercise outside of the clinical setting *while asymptomatic*. The aim of the second stage of the treatment hierarchy is to make the exercises automatic, and to ensure that the vocal folds are in the optimum position at rest. Intensive practice during asymptomatic periods is required to maximise motor learning and will eventually facilitate rapid recall and initiation of the exercises during symptomatic periods. A sufficient number of repetitions are necessary. The patient should perform the breathing exercises frequently throughout the day when asymptomatic, for example, five breath sequences on 20 separate occasions during the day or ten breath sequences on ten separate occasions.

The speech pathologist and patient can identify appropriate times to complete these exercises. Key times may be on waking but before rising from bed, after rising from bed, while waiting for water in the shower to warm up, while waiting for the kettle to boil, before inhaled medications, while waiting for the computer to load, before periods of physical activity, while reading the newspaper, while waiting in line, when on hold on the telephone. The exercises should also be completed in a variety of body positions including standing, sitting, bending over, while doing housework, and walking. The posture that the patient is most likely to be using throughout the day, for example bending over a sewing machine or on a bicycle, should be incorporated into the practice schedule. The exercises should be performed even when the patient is feeling well. Many patients report that they like to perform the exercises while driving the car. While this is a good opportunity to optimise time, care should be taken to ensure that the car is not the only time the exercise is performed. The car does not allow for optimal body posture and the individual is likely to be distracted.

The third stage in the treatment hierarchy is for the patient to use the technique outside the clinical setting during *symptomatic* periods to prevent, or interrupt the cough or respiratory symptoms. In order to do this, the patient needs to recognise when a cough is about to occur and then substitute the cough suppression exercise as a competing response to cough. The speech pathologist may need to encourage the patient to become familiar with the precipitating sensation of the urge to cough – no matter how faint. The patient is encouraged to continue the technique until they feel safe and comfortable again. Patients should also do their cough suppression exercise before situations where they are likely to be at risk, for example, before physical exercise. If the patient is avoiding social situations, such as attending movies, lectures or meetings, encourage them to sit close to an exit so they can leave quickly, gain control over their symptoms and then return to that situation.[1]

The final stage of the treatment hierarchy involves deliberately exposing the patient to identified triggers such as exertion, or other irritants. The patient performs the cough suppression technique, then applies a brief exposure while continuing to utilise the technique to inhibit their symptoms, and continues to use the exercises after the exposure has ceased. For example, if cold air is a known trigger for cough, the patient can perform their cough suppression exercise and then deliberately expose themselves to cold air for a specified period of time, while still performing the cough suppression exercise. This exposure could be achieved by opening a refrigerator or walking into an air-conditioned building. Alternatively, if perfume is identified as a trigger to cough, the patient can perform the cough suppression exercise, then deliberately expose themselves to perfume while continuing to perform the cough suppression exercise. With exertion, begin the technique before the physical exercise and for the duration of the exercise. Exercise intensity should be reduced immediately at the very first sign of tightness or irritation, but increased as the patient tolerates with no symptoms. The initial exposure time can be short, for example 30 seconds, and gradually increase in duration as tolerated by the patient.

Although there are a number of cough suppression techniques available, it is important to start with one technique, rather than present several techniques at once. Patients are more likely to perform the technique accurately and adhere to therapy recommendations if they are achievable and not excessive.

Distraction techniques

Distraction techniques include sipping water, sucking on ice chips, chewing gum, sucking non-medicated lollipops, or waiting for 5 to 10 seconds to see whether the urge to cough passes. These techniques may be sufficient to suppress mild throat clearing, or to incorporate into the management of cough towards the end of therapy. In isolation, they are rarely sufficient to suppress cough in the initial stages of therapy.

Posture

Body position is very important when doing the paradoxical vocal fold movement release and cough suppression exercises. Patients may need to change their motor pattern so that they respond to incoming stimuli in a manner which is not harmful. Stemple[5] advises frequent monitoring of body tension throughout the day, and exhaling frequently throughout the day. The patient may sit with their back well-supported and release tension in their shoulders. If needed, they can start in a semi-supine position and eventually move upright in order to increase abdominal movement. When proficient, they can practice the exercises during walking, running or other aerobic activity.

The speech pathologist should be cognisant of the way in which they instruct the patient regarding their posture. The instructions given to patients during voice therapy are applicable to the treatment of cough and paradoxical vocal fold movement. Patients are more likely to retain instructions when they can explore their own posture and movement, rather than hear an implicit verbal instruction. For example, rather than say *"lower your shoulders"* or *"sit up straight"*, say *"notice whether there is any tension in your shoulders"* or *"notice whether your weight is evenly distributed between your two feet and two hips when sitting"*. These latter instructions enable the patient to explore their own posture. While this process takes longer giving an implicit instruction, it enables the patient to recall the posture at a later time. If the invitation to adjust posture is not helpful, then the speech pathologist can apply physical guidance of neck, head, shoulder and body posture, and invite the patient to notice the difference.[6] In addition to focusing on posture, it is also helpful to have the patient place their hand on the lower abdominal muscles to monitor abdominal movement during respiration and notice the lower abdominal movement.

Cough suppression swallow

The cough suppression swallow is a technique that is ideal for supressing throat clearing and coughing that has a deliberate component. This technique has the advantage that it is easy to use and can be taught quickly in the clinical setting. For some patients, this technique alone is sufficient to gain control of cough symptoms (see Appendix 9).

To perform this technique, the patient is instructed to combine an effortful swallow with a Valsalva manoeuvre, combined with an isometric push, similar to that used in the treatment of oropharyngeal dysphagia,[7] and with the head in a flexed position (Figure 9.1). The technique can be performed as a dry swallow, or in combination with sipping water or sucking on a non-medicated lozenge. The technique is performed at the very first sign of irritation or the urge to cough. The speech pathologist should ensure that the patient is pushing their hands toward each other, rather than onto their abdomen, while performing this technique. This exercise is easily modified for use in public by removing the hand movement. Although this exercise is quick and easy to learn, it is not always effective in reducing the urge to cough, and other cough control breathing techniques may be required.

Cough control breathing

The goal of cough control breathing* is to prevent or interrupt the cough by using a breathing technique designed to inhibit vocal fold adduction and maintain vocal fold abduction throughout the breathing cycle. To commence this exercise, the patient is seated and instructed to breathe in and out, while monitoring their breathing. Monitoring may involve feeling the movement of the lower abdominal muscles during respiration, or alternatively, monitoring oral or nasal airflow on their hand or finger.

The patient should then take a gentle breath in, ideally through their nose, and then blow out quickly through very tight lips. The tight sphincter of the lips is used to replace the narrow sphincter of the larynx during cough. This exercise creates a strong thrust of air which is designed to mimic the rapid speed of air through the larynx during cough. This airstream gives the sensation of blowing out what is experienced as obstructing the airway. The patient is encouraged to sense the same degree of work during this exercise as when they cough. Tightness and excessive effort during inhalation needs to be avoided to prevent triggering another cough.

The speech pathologist can explore different breathing patterns with the patient during this exercise. These patterns can include changes to the method

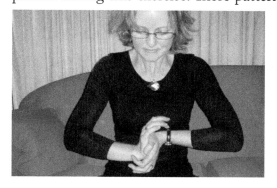

Figure 9.1: Cough suppression swallow technique.

of inhalation or exhalation, as well as changes to the breathing rhythm. The patient can breathe in through their nose or mouth, or alternatively, sniff to abduct the vocal folds. Another alternative is breathing in and out through tightly pursed lips, while listening to the sound of the air passing.. During exhalation, the patient may blow out through pursed lips,

---

* This therapy has been adapted from a handout by Fran Lowry, National Jewish Medical & Research Centre, Denver, Colorado, USA.

blow on to a finger in order to sense the expired air, or exhale onto a voiceless fricative sound. The breathing rhythm can also be altered so that inhalation and exhalation are of equal time, either short or long, or short inhalation and long exhalation. Many patients have more difficulty with the inhalation than the exhalation component of this exercise.

Once the patient can perform the technique accurately in the clinical setting, they need to practice it frequently during asymptomatic periods so that it becomes automatic, for example five repetitions, 20 times a day. Once they can perform the technique accurately, they can use it to prevent or interrupt the cough in daily situations. They will need to become aware of the sensation or urge to cough that precipitates the cough, and start to use the cough control breathing technique immediately.

Some patients will be unable to prevent the cough and may need to be coached to interrupt or reduce the severity of cough episodes. For example, they could be guided to shorten the duration of the coughing episode. This process requires considerable energy and patients may need reassurance to continue. The speech pathologist may need to work alongside the patient to coach them into cutting off the end of the cough.[1]

Cough control breathing can be used as a preventative strategy in situations where patients are more vulnerable or at risk of coughing,[1] such as first thing in the morning, while bending over, or in the supermarket. This breathing pattern should be maintained for the duration of the exposure. The patient may require reassurance that they are not a failure if a cough breaks through during these situations. In extreme cases, the speech pathologist may explore the use of codeine or cough suppressants with the medical officer to suppress the cough initially, and then institute behavioural management.

Throat clearing control

Some patients present with throat clearing rather than coughing, or may present with a combination of throat clearing and coughing. Patients with cough associated with other diseases, such as bronchiectasis or chronic obstructive pulmonary disease, may present with persistent throat clearing in combination with a productive cough. The aim of the therapy for chronic throat clearing is to eliminate throat clearing by substituting a tight, effortful swallow.[*]

The first stage of throat clearing control is for the patient to understand that throat clearing occurs because of an irritation in the throat, although often in the absence of a physical need to clear the throat. Throat clearing is a phonotraumatic behaviour which, while performed to relieve irritation, can actually cause further irritation. This pattern eventually becomes habitual and can occur subconsciously. The program is only effective if the patient gives it their attention and follows the required steps. This might mean that the patient makes the throat clearing suppression their highest priority for several days.

The first step in the throat clearing control program is to raise the patient's awareness of the frequency of their throat clearing. This is achieved by having the patient record each throat clearing episode in a diary. The speech pathologist or family member may need to draw the patient's attention to each throat clearing episode initially. At this stage, the patient will become aware of their throat clearing *after* the event but not before.

Each time the patient notices their throat clearing, they should perform an effortful swallow of either saliva or a small quantity of water and record in their diary. These steps increase the patient's awareness of the frequency of their throat clearing. Patients may need several prompts to follow this sequence in the clinical setting. Many patients remark that they are unaware of the extent to which they clear their throat at this stage in the therapy.

After one or two days, the patient may become aware that they are throat clearing during the throat clearing episode. They should be encouraged to perform the effortful swallow and record each throat clearing episode in their diary.

After a further two days, it is hoped that the patient will become aware of the urge before they actually throat clear. At this stage they should be able to do the effortful swallow instead of throat clearing.

PVFM-release breathing

PVFM-release breathing is also known as *Breathing Exercises for VCD* or *Relaxed Throat Breathing*. Some might consider them separate exercises, and there are certainly variations on components of the exercise. PVFM-release exercises[8] can

---

[*] This therapy program has been adapted from a handout by Fran Lowry, National Jewish Medical & Research Centre, Denver, Colorado, USA.

be initiated during inhalation or exhalation. Tension should be released in the upper body, shoulders and neck during inhalation. Jaw or temporomandibular joint tension should be monitored. Inhalation should occur with the tongue released on the floor of the mouth. The lips should be gently closed or relaxed.

The patient inhales while noticing the abdominal muscles relax and fill through the middle. Upper chest movement should be minimal, but does not need to be absent. To engage the lower abdominal muscles, encourage the patient to stand and place their thumb in their navel and rest the remaining fingers against the lower abdominal muscles. Encourage the patient to *notice* the lower abdominal movement and an easy rhythm, rather than force the movement. Newsham[9] recommends bending at the waist, crouching, or kneeling to promote diaphragmatic breathing. The speed of inhalation and exhalation can be altered while maintaining focus on the abdomen.

Inhalation

Several inhalation methods can be used in PVFM-release breathing. Inhalation can occur with pursed lips, or by nasal breathing and closed lips to open the vocal folds. Alternatively, sniffing has the advantage of contracting the posterior cricoarytenoid muscle, which abducts the vocal folds. The pattern chosen will vary depending on what feels easiest for the individual patient. Patients are encouraged to breathe in the amount of air that feels natural, rather than taking a large breath. Stemple[2] suggests that large inhalation promotes tension as the patient has to attempt to retain all the air. Patients are encouraged to exhale what they inhale rather than retaining air. Some patients may be reluctant to let go of all their air as they are worried that they will be unable to inspire any more air. There should be no breath holding immediately after the inhalation.

Using the sniffing technique many times a day may also help to reprogram the system.[2] The sniff should occur with the mouth closed and there should be no breath hold immediately after the sniff. Another inhalation method is the *reverse candle blow*.[1] In this technique, the patient mimes blowing out a candle and then while maintaining the same lip position, 'sips' back the same air that was exhaled during the blow. The reverse candle blow encourages gentle inhalation without breath holding, laryngeal constriction, or excess effort. Inhaling through a straw helps to regulate the amount of air inspired and promotes constriction at the lips rather than the larynx.

Inhalation should last for approximately one second, but this inhalation time is simply a guide. In practice, it is more important for the patient to focus on relaxed inhalation, rather than make the inhalation last for a pre-specified period of time.

Exhalation

Exhalation should occur with a relaxed mouth, through gently pursed lips. Some patients may prefer to exhale on a gentle /f/, /s/, /ʃ/, a lazy breath out, effortless exhale, breathing out through a straw or through tightly pursed lips. The choice of position will vary according to patient preference and the patient will develop an exhalation pattern that they feel comfortable using the majority of the time. Some patients may like to adopt an alternative posture in public to that which they do at home, such as using gentle pursed lips or exhaling on /f/.

The patient should breathe out to an extent that feels comfortable, but they do not need to exhale all their air. Exhalation should last for approximately three seconds but may be varied as the patient becomes more confident. These expiratory manoeuvres are designed to create some resistance to the expired breath stream. This process reduces the speed of airflow exiting from the oral cavity, which increases the volume of air in the oral cavity. The air pressure is subsequently increased in the oral cavity and pharynx which, in turn, promotes vocal fold abduction. Some patients benefit from the explanation of the physiology behind this process in order to appreciate that there is a scientific basis for the exercise.

Both inhalation and exhalation should be easy and they should occur together in an easy rhythm with no breath-holding in between. The patient should not have to pull to get air in or push to get air out. They should notice abdominal muscles move in and out, but not force. Patients may need encouragement to slow down and make the breathing natural. PVFM-release breathing can feel foreign to patients initially. Patients may be used to rapid, noisy or effortful breathing with repeated attempts to compensate for their respiratory difficulty. Therapy aims to recalibrate the patient's perception of an efficient and effortless respiratory system.

PVFM-release breathing can be adapted to prevent coughing episodes, particularly if the patient feels that deep breathing triggers cough. The patient identifies which part of the body the cough is coming from and breathes to that point.[8] Care must be taken to maintain abdominal movement during respiration and avoid shoulder tension.

Murry[10] describes the respiratory retraining technique which is very similar to PVFM-release breathing. This technique involves four stages and is described in details in Chapter 11. The first stage is quiet rhythmic breathing where the patient is encouraged to exhale with relaxed shoulders and abdominal movement. Patients are then instructed to exhale while sustaining a prolonged fricative, such as /ʃ/, /f/, or /s/, for increasing lengths of time. The patient then performs pulsed exhalation where they are instructed to produce a pulse of air using /ha/ or /ʃa/, followed by sniffing through the nose with the mouth closed. There is also an abdominal focus at rest where patient lies supine, focusing on abdominal movement during inspiration and expiration. Once this is achieved, the patient can breathe through resistance such as a straw whilst maintaining the abdominal focus.

Once the patient can perform PVFM-release breathing accurately in the clinical setting, they are encouraged to practice frequently at home during asymptomatic periods, for example five repetitions, 20 times a day. The purpose of this practice is to facilitate rapid recall of the exercise at the very first sign of breathing difficulty or urge to cough. Once the technique is automatic, it can be used at the first sense of throat tightness or breathing difficulty with the aim of preventing or suppressing paradoxical vocal fold movement episodes. The exercise should also be performed before taking any asthma medication.

Emergency strategies for paradoxical vocal fold movement

Patients who experience severe paradoxical vocal fold movement episodes need a strategy to quickly release from the episodes. Severe paradoxical vocal fold movement episodes may be accompanied by a sense of panic, which increases laryngeal tension and anxiety. Some patients may even call an ambulance or present to the emergency department during an acute episode. If the patient has a history of severe and frightening episodes, it is necessary for them to have an action plan in place that they can implement in case of an emergency.

The action plan should be simple and easy to recall. The aim is to change the patient's breathing pattern and give them immediate control over their breathing. The strategies will eventually provide the patient with more confidence about actively managing their breathing, rather than passively experiencing breathing difficulties.

Several different breathing strategies may be used for emergency situations. Some patients may simply be able to use their PVFM-release exercises in response to severe paradoxical vocal fold movement episodes. Others might be able to reduce their respiratory rate, relax and concentrate on nasal breathing, sniffing or breathing through a straw. Alternatively, the patient can be taught a specific sequence of breathing techniques to follow. For example, the patient sniffs to abduct the vocal folds, then breathes out through tightly pursed lips to maintain vocal fold abduction. The patient does five of these breaths, takes a sip of water and then repeats the whole sequence five times. Counting the repetitions can serve to distract the patient from the fact that their breathing is difficult. Attention needs to be paid to ensuring that the mouth is closed, that there is no clavicular movement and that there is no excess force of effort during inhalation. The patient should refrain from talking, while attempting to release paradoxical vocal fold movement in order to concentrate on their breathing. The exact exercise pattern can be varied according to what is most comfortable for the patient.

The plan should be documented in a way that is helpful for the patient to access easily. The example in Figure 9.2 is designed for the person to carry with them in their phone, wallet or noticeboard so that it is easily accessible in several places. The emergency management plan for patients with combined paradoxical vocal fold movement and asthma can be incorporated into the same document, in consultation with the respiratory physician.

Emergency Strategies for PVFM	Emergency Strategies for combined PVFM and asthma
1. Sniff. 2. Blow out through pursed lips. 3. Repeat 5 times. 4. Sip water. Continue this sequence five times. Then continue your exercises.	1. Breathe in and out though a straw. 2. PVFM-Release exercises. 3. Take asthma inhaler. 4. Continue straw breathing or PVFM-Release breathing. 5. Sip water.

Figure 9.2: Examples of emergency strategies for paradoxical vocal fold movement.

PVFM-release during physical exercise

PVFM-release breathing exercises can be modified to use during intense physical activity. The patient needs to establish good technique with the PVFM-release exercises initially, which may require one or two therapy sessions. Once the patient can perform the PVFM-release exercises accurately, they can incorporate them into physical activity.

The patient begins by doing the PVFM-release breathing at rest, and then while doing gentle physical exercise, such as walking on the spot, walking slowly across a room, or performing repeated arm raises. They are coached to pay attention to their breathing and, in particular, the ease of their breathing. If their breathing remains easy the intensity of the physical exercise can be increased. The intensity of the exercise will depend to some extent on the degree of physical fitness. However, if breathing becomes difficult or tightness is noted, the patient should decrease the intensity of the physical exercise. This process is in contrast to the typical pattern of physical exercise where breathing is automatically adjusted to accommodate exercise intensity. Patients often need encouragement to reduce their exercise intensity. The pattern of breathing can change slightly with increased physical exercise. Some patients may find it easier to focus their breathing on their rib cage rather than the lower abdomen, particularly during more intense exercise such as running.

In addition to adjusting exercise intensity, the timing of exhalation may need to change so that it occurs during the most strenuous part of the exercise. For example, when lifting weights, inhale while releasing the weight and exhale while lifting the weight. This sequence is often counter intuitive and requires ongoing reinforcement by the speech pathologist.

Laryngeal deconstriction

Laryngeal deconstriction techniques were traditionally developed for the treatment of dysphonia. Laryngeal constriction is first released during respiration and then the released posture is maintained during phonation. The aim of this process in voice therapy is to fully retract the false vocal folds during phonation in order to allow the true vocal folds to vibrate unimpeded.

Some patients with chronic refractory cough may subconsciously constrict their vocal folds during respiration as a compensatory reaction to laryngeal irritation. This pattern can be particularly prevalent in patients with previous irritant exposure who are fearful of repeated injury and who have a tendency to over-protect their airway. These patients may benefit from therapy to incorporate laryngeal deconstriction exercises into respiration and phonation.

Laryngeal deconstriction exercises for the treatment of dysphonia are familiar to most speech pathologists. Techniques, such as the *silent giggle*, are described in the Estill and Voicecraft programs. Constriction can be released by inviting the patient to compare the sound produced when taking in a deep breath to the sound produced when taking in a silent breath. Noisy inspiration is usually associated increased tension in the vocal folds and the vocal folds may not be fully abducted. Negative practice can be used during this exercise to increase awareness of the contrast between constricted and released laryngeal posture.

In chronic refractory cough and paradoxical vocal fold movement, these exercises may be adapted to having the patient increase their conscious awareness of constriction. For example, the patient may deliberately constrict their vocal folds by holding their breath followed by releasing constriction while contrasting the differences in sensation between constricted and abducted vocal folds. Once the task can be performed at rest, the complexity can be increased to include maintaining the correct posture during movement and speech. Laryngeal deconstriction can also be used to promote a sense of control over laryngeal function during respiration. This can increase awareness of any tension in the larynx during respiration and contrast it with the laryngeal sensation when the tension is released.[9]

Respiratory muscle training devices

Respiratory muscle strength training devices can target either inspiratory or expiratory function, and aim to strengthen the inspiratory and expiratory muscles. Resistive trainers are affected by the patient's breathing rate. In pressure threshold devices, patients must overcome threshold load by generating sufficient inspiratory pressure. Respiratory muscle training devices may be useful for patients with chronic refractory cough and paradoxical vocal fold movement.

Mathers-Schmidt and Brilla[11] reported a case study of inspiratory muscle training in a single case study of an athlete with exercise-induced paradoxical vocal fold movement. This therapy program differed from earlier behavioural treatment programs for paradoxical vocal fold movement. It involved daily training sessions over a ten-week period, whereby the participant inhaled against resistance. Treatment resulted in reduced glottal closure during inspiration, and elimination of paradoxical vocal fold movement symptoms during strenuous exercise.

Modified Accent Method Breathing

The modified Accent Method Breathing technique was traditionally used in treatment of dysphonia and has been adapted for both singing training and speech pathology. This technique aims to increase pulmonary output while reducing laryngeal muscle tension during phonation.[5] The theory is that strong subglottal air pressure will increase the amplitude of vocal fold vibration and improve the stability of the closed phase of vocal fold vibration. This technique can also be adapted in the treatment of chronic refractory cough and paradoxical vocal fold movement. In this technique, the patient stands with their fingers resting on their lower abdominal muscles (see Figure 9.3) and notices the movement of those muscles during the voice exercises. Voiceless fricative sounds are performed initially and voiced fricatives are introduced once voiceless sounds are mastered. The patient sustains a single sound alternating with the speech pathologist, while focusing on lower abdominal muscles and maintaining a rhythm. The exercises are performed with a metronome set at 55 beats per minute and 3 beats per bar or measure, and each sound is sustained for approximately 3 beats. Numerous apps and online metronomes can be used for this purpose. Other rhythms described in the Accent Method Breathing treatment program can also be used, however it is our experience that single exhalations are usually adequate for the patient to gain control over their respiratory muscles.

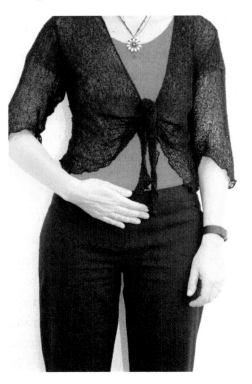

Figure 9.3: Example of noticing movement in the lower abdominal muscles. The thumb rests in the navel with the remaining fingers feeling the movement of the lower abdominal muscles.

Reducing laryngeal irritation

Reducing laryngeal irritation is largely based on vocal hygiene training. Most speech pathologists are familiar with the concepts of vocal hygiene training as this is a critical component in many voice therapy programs. The emphasis in reducing laryngeal irritation includes reducing laryngeal irritants, desensitisation, improving hydration and reducing phonotrauma. A handout for patients is included in Appendix 10. In order to facilitate patient adherence to vocal hygiene advice, it is recommended that the pertinent information for each patient is highlighted rather than giving the patient the entire list of recommendations.

Reduce laryngeal irritants

The first component of vocal hygiene training in the treatment of chronic refractory cough is to reduce laryngeal irritation that may exacerbate cough. Most patients with chronic refractory cough report exposure to laryngeal irritants. The role of the speech pathologist is to educate the patient regarding the effects of these irritants on cough and laryngeal function and problem-solve strategies for the patient.

1. **Avoid or reduce alcohol.** It would be ideal to avoid alcohol. It may be possible to negotiate eliminating alcohol for a specified period of time, for example two months, and then gradually reintroduce it once symptoms are under control. For patients who do not feel it is possible to avoid alcohol, reducing the quantity and frequency of alcohol consumption, or alternating alcoholic and non-alcoholic beverages might be a helpful compromise.

2. **Avoid smoking.** Smoking is a leading cause of laryngeal cancer and pathology. Few patients referred for behavioural treatment of cough smoke. However if patients do smoke a referral for smoking cessation may be required.

3. **Avoid or reduce caffeine.** Caffeine can cause irritation to the vocal folds and can also exacerbate reflux that triggers cough. Reducing or eliminating caffeine can reduce laryngeal irritation and cough. Vocal hygiene programs commonly recommend reducing or eliminating caffeine as it affects systemic hydration. Erickson-Levendoski[12] studied the effects of caffeine consumption on phonation threshold pressure and perceived phonatory effort during a vocal loading task in 16 healthy individuals

aged 18–32 years. The participants in this study had equivalent of 24 oz, or 750 ml of coffee. There were no significant differences in phonation threshold pressure or perceived phonatory effort between caffeine or sham conditions. The authors speculated that healthy individuals might compensate for the diuretic effects of caffeine. Although caffeine did not appear to affect voice measures in healthy controls in this study, the effect of caffeine on individuals with dysphonia, laryngeal hypersensitivity, or chronic refractory cough remains unclear. Furthermore, the effect of caffeine on older individuals or higher doses of caffeine remains unknown. Perhaps it is sufficient to avoid excessive caffeine consumption rather than eliminate it entirely.

4. **Promote nasal breathing.** Nasal breathing reduces the irritating effect of dry cold air on the larynx. While it is difficult to change habitual breathing patterns, the speech pathologist can monitor nasal versus mouth breathing during therapy sessions. Once the patient is aware of their breathing route, they can attempt nasal breathing for short periods of time, while continuously monitoring their breathing. They can then attempt nasal breathing for gradually increasing periods of time.

5. **Avoid medicated cough lozenges.** Many patients with chronic refractory cough consume medicated cough lozenges even though recognizing that they do not have a beneficial effect their cough. Long term use of medicated cough lozenges is often not recommended due to the drying effect of ingredients such as menthol and the anesthetic properties that reduce awareness of phonotrauma and subsequent damage. However, further research about the long term effects of cough lozenges in chronic refractory cough is required.

6. **Behavioural management of reflux.** Behavioural management of reflux is critical and is described in more detail in Chapter 10. It is our experience that few patients actively incorporate behavioural management of reflux, despite being given previous advice by their doctor. The speech pathologist has an important role in supporting the patient with lifestyle management of reflux.

Desensitisation

A formal desensitisation program may be required for some patients, particularly if they believe they are allergic to particular substances. Desensitisation should be performed in consultation with the patient's physician. Some patients may need to disinvest their notion of an allergy to certain substances. Some sensitivities occur in response to harmless environmental stimuli which are perceived as harmful to the airway and, when exposed, lead to symptoms of cough and paradoxical vocal fold movement.

Irritant challenges involve exposing patients to a known trigger with the aim of controlling the symptoms despite exposure to the trigger. Although the ultimate aim is to have the patient avoid symptoms, in the initial stages they may also need to learn how to interrupt or abort an episode when exposed to the irritant.

The following component of the program has been adapted from Milner[13] and may be suitable for patients with cough and paradoxical vocal fold movement symptoms associated with specific irritants. The first step is to have the patient list the specific irritants and order them from least to most difficult. Prior to exposing the patient to the irritant, the patient commences their breathing exercises: for example, the cough control breathing or paradoxical vocal fold movement release breathing. This is where excellent technique is important.

The patient is then exposed to a very small amount of the irritant for a controlled period of time. For example, if the patient is irritated by garlic odour or perfume, a small amount is placed into a cup with a lid that can easily be removed and replaced. The patient performs exercises while exposed to the irritant. The exposure time is controlled and gradually increased once the patient gains control of their symptoms. The initial exposure time should be short even if the patient does not experience any difficulty. If the patient does experience difficulty the irritant should be removed.

The goal of desensitisation is for the patient to tolerate longer periods of exposure to the irritant. Some patients require a cue from the speech pathologist to use the breathing techniques when they start to notice symptoms. This cueing is particularly necessary for patients who have an external locus of control, i.e. those that perceive the irritant is causing the symptom, rather than viewing the symptoms as a behavioural response to the irritant. The speech pathologist will need to remind the patient to implement the breathing exercises to recover if they experience difficulty, and to avoid maladaptive patterns such as breath holding, poor posture and shallow breathing. A nose clip (Figure 9.4) may be used to promote oral breathing initially and allow the patient to control their symptoms while exposed to the irritant. It reduces the impact of the odour on the respiratory response.

Once the patient has mastered irritant exposure in the clinical setting with the speech pathologist, they may start to coordinate their own controlled exposures outside of the clinical setting. For example, the patient sets up their own exposures to perfumes and cleaning products at home, or go to environments such as shopping centres where there is an increased likelihood of exposure. Over time, it is anticipated that the patient will learn to prevent and control their symptoms and that they will eventually become less sensitive to common irritants.

Hydration

The third component of vocal hygiene training aims to improve both surface and systemic hydration. Many patients with chronic refractory cough are poorly hydrated. Strategies for improving surface and systemic hydration in chronic refractory cough are similar to those used in the treatment of hyperfunctional voice disorders.

Systemic hydration involves hydration of the whole body. Fluids are absorbed by intestinal cells, transferred to the capillary network and transported around the body by the vascular system.[14] Homeostatic mechanisms maintain precise regulation of water balance and exist at both cellular and whole body levels.[15] Adequate systemic hydration reduces the phonation threshold pressure.[16]

Two litres of water a day is often recommended to maintain adequate systemic hydration however, further studies are needed to confirm the actual amount of water required.[15] Patients may require more water if they are talking extensively, exercising, or in hot weather. The frequency of water drinking also needs to increase. Frequent sips of water throughout the day can have a greater effect on the urge to cough than the same volume consumed less

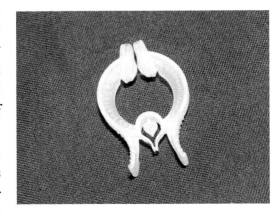

Figure 9.4: A nose clip can be used to prevent nasal breathing during irritant exposure and reduce the impact of odour on the respiratory response.

frequently. Flavouring with fruit, small quantities of juice or mint leaves can make the water more palatable.

Drinking water can be helpful to suppress coughing or throat clearing episodes. A single sip of water may be insufficient to prevent a coughing episode if it associated with significant laryngeal irritation. In some situations, the individual may need to consume half to one whole cup of water in order to relieve the symptoms.

Surface hydration refers to moisture levels on the epithelial surface of the vocal folds.[14] Adequate surface hydration can reduce vocal effort. It is targeted through steam inhalation. The patient is simply advised to inhale steam without adding anything to the water. It should be noted, however, that some patients find steam may trigger their cough and recommendations may need to be tailored to specific individuals. Various commercial devices for steam inhalation may be used. Alternatively, filling a sink with boiling water or an inverted funnel placed over a cup of boiling water are cost effective methods. Inhaling steam during the shower may be less intense, but easier for patients to complete on a regular basis.

Although not classified as hydration, strategies to increase the frequency of swallowing can reduce the sensation of laryngeal irritation. It is hypothesised that swallowing temporarily reduces cough reflex sensitivity. Swallow frequency can be increased by sucking (not chewing) on non-medicated lozenges, chewing gum or swallowing whole teaspoons of honey. Paul *et al.*[17] found that swallowing teaspoons of honey was an effective treatment for acute cough in paediatric patients. This study compared the effects of honey, or honey-flavoured dextromethorphan with no treatment on acute nocturnal cough in children with upper respiratory tract infections. Honey was rated most favourably in reducing cough and improving sleep. Paul concluded that honey may be a preferable treatment for the cough and sleep difficulty associated with childhood upper respiratory tract infection. Although not studied in patients with chronic refractory cough, it is hypothesised that the sticky properties of honey result in frequent swallowing which again might reduce cough sensitivity.

Reducing phonotraumatic behaviours

Phonotraumatic vocal behaviours may exacerbate laryngeal irritation and contribute to the cough. These may need to be addressed as part of the therapy program. Some of these behaviours may require a more formal course of voice therapy, whereas others may be addressed simultaneously with the cough suppression techniques. For example, a patient who habitually clears their throat prior to initiating phonation may simply need their attention drawn to the behaviour, whereas a patient who is using a laryngeal focus of resonance may require resonant voice therapy.

Phonotraumatic vocal behaviours may need to be targeted in therapy if their phonatory pattern contributes to laryngeal irritation, even if the patient is unconcerned about their voice. Minimisation of phonotraumatic behaviours during phonation, such as hard glottal attacks, speaking at inappropriate pitch or loudness level, speaking on residual air, or speaking with excessive laryngeal tension, is required. Shulman[2] suggests other strategies including speaking from a yawn position, rather than a swallow position, and to speak from the tip of the tongue. This suggests reducing laryngeal constriction and laryngeal focus of resonance. Shulman[2] also describes tongue placement exercises to increase tongue tip control and flexibility. Therapy includes repetition of single sounds, words and short sentences with anterior tongue placement emphasising the easy onset of sound.

Voice therapy techniques such as resonant voice therapy[6] might also be included in the treatment program. This technique is particularly helpful for patients who report that talking triggers cough. Resonant voice therapy reduces vocal fold impact stress during phonation. There is also preliminary evidence that resonant voice therapy might reduce inflammation triggered by vocal loading.[18] Nevertheless, resonant voice therapy promotes a more efficient pattern of phonation which is likely to reduce irritation leading to coughing.

The larynx has a physiological limit that varies from time to time and from person to person.[13] The degree of talking that results in vocal fatigue varies between individuals. Talking with strain and excess effort during periods of upper respiratory tract infection can exacerbate dysphonia and may need to be modified during therapy. Likewise, yelling, screaming and prolonged loud talking contribute to phonotrauma if the correct technique is not used.

Psychoeducational counselling

Psychoeducational counselling is the final component of the speech pathology program for chronic refractory cough. The effectiveness of speech pathology treatment very much depends upon patient adherence to the treatment program. The aim of psychoeducational counselling is to increase adherence and motivation for the behavioural management program. This component of therapy may be delivered in discrete therapy sessions, or it may be interspersed throughout the program through supportive comments. Some speech pathologists may prefer to take the patient's lead when delivering this component of the program.

Many of the recommendations and suggestions given to patients in therapy might appear to contradict with their beliefs or advice given by other health professionals. Patients may need support to relinquish previously held beliefs about their cough and the strategies they have used for their cough. Patients should feel safe to ask questions and raise objections throughout the course of therapy.

The concepts of motivational interviewing are particularly important in the treatment of chronic refractory cough. Motivational interviewing is a semi-directive client-centred counselling style for eliciting behaviour change by helping clients explore and resolve ambivalence.[19] Motivational interviewing aims to engage the patient's intrinsic motivation to change their behaviour. The four components of motivational interviewing are expressing empathy, developing discrepancy, rolling with resistance and supporting self-efficacy.[19]

Express empathy

The speech pathologist can assist the patient to share their experiences in a non-judgmental manner by asking open ended questions and teasing out information. The aim is to understand the situation from the patient's point of view, even if the patient says something that is scientifically incorrect. An accurate understanding of the patient's experience may help to facilitate change.[20] Patients with chronic refractory cough may feel frustration that others have not understood their symptoms, or may be fearful about the severity of their symptoms. The speech pathologist will also need to support the patient regarding any fear surrounding respiration, particularly if there has been a history of cough syncope or associated paradoxical vocal fold movement. Patients may feel that they are going to die during these severe episodes. The speech pathologist needs to demonstrate empathy and understanding of the problem, while still establishing the need for the patient to follow the recommended strategies. Expressing empathy will facilitate engagement in the therapy process. Many patients have consulted other health professionals and other individuals before being referred to the speech pathologist. Advice received from these sources may conflict with the speech pathology advice, may indicate that the symptoms cannot be explained, or that treatment is unlikely to be successful.[2] The patient should feel confident that the speech pathologist understands their interpretation of these issues relating to their cough.

The speech pathologist may need to assist the patient to relinquish a medical diagnosis or the search for the cause of their cough. This can be achieved by validating the patient's concerns about their cough, and understanding the impact of cough on their quality of life and their frustration at the protracted course of medical investigation and treatment for their cough. Patients often require acknowledgement that their perception of the urge to cough is real, but that the need to cough is not.[1]

Develop discrepancy

Developing discrepancy is useful when the patient says they want to do one thing, but then does another. The speech pathologist's task here is to identify the discrepancy and bring it to the fore. The patient may be unaware of the discrepancy until it is highlighted by the clinician. For example, a patient may be very frustrated by their cough and want to gain control, but then forget to practice their exercises, or not use their exercises to interrupt or prevent the coughing episodes. In this case, the speech pathologist could point out this discrepancy to the patient. For example, *"So can I clarify that I understand this correctly – on one hand you are bothered by your cough and want it to stop, but then you find it hard to remember to practice your exercises and hard to remember to use your exercises to stop yourself coughing. I wonder why that is the case"*. The speech pathologist and patient can then discuss and examine the discrepancies between their current behaviour and their future health goals. The speech pathologist can help the patient to problem solve strategies to reach their goal. The patient is more likely to be motivated to change their behaviour once they perceive that their current behaviour is not congruent with their treatment goals.

Roll with resistance

Rolling with resistance is preferred to confronting the patient about their resistance to therapy recommendations. The patient is encouraged to develop solutions to the problems that they have identified. Reinforcing arguments is unhelpful in the therapeutic process. For example, if a patient says it is impossible to stop coughing, the speech pathologist may ask permission to share research evidence about the role of the cerebral cortex during cough. For example,

"That's interesting that you say that. Would you like me to tell you about some of the newer research into the brain's ability to control cough?"

Support self-efficacy

Supporting self-efficacy is aimed at helping the patient develop the belief that they are able to achieve change. Rewarding small behaviour changes and gains is extremely beneficial. One strategy is to ask the patient to rate their motivation to change on a scale of 1 to 10, and then ask the patient what it would take to move them from the number they have rated to a higher number. For example, *"So on a scale of 1 to 10, how important is it for you to use the exercises to stop your coughing episodes?"* If the patient answers *"Five..."*, *"That's great. What would it take for you to move to a seven?"* This process helps the patient to own their personal changes.

Emotional issues

Some patients report that emotional issues can be a trigger for the cough and paradoxical vocal fold movement symptoms. These patients will require additional support to respond to emotional issues in a different way. Often, simply acknowledging emotional issues as a trigger can be sufficient for some patients.

In more serious cases, patients may need referral to a mental health professional. Time may need to be invested in preparing the patient for referral. Cognitive behavioural therapy may be needed to address anticipated anxiety or the repressed vocal expression of emotions that subsequently trigger the cough and respiratory symptoms.[2]

Some patients also require assistance to develop realistic expectations about their progress in therapy. They may need to appreciate that therapy is hard work and that intensive practice may be needed to achieve therapy gains. Symptoms are unlikely to completely resolve overnight and it may take several weeks or months for the patient to develop control. A realistic goal for some patients is control over, rather than full elimination of their cough.

Summary

Speech pathology intervention for chronic refractory cough involves several components. Education is required to facilitate acceptance of the behavioural management program - particularly that cough is not necessary and that there is potential for voluntary control over cough. Symptom control techniques are designed as a substitute for cough. The patient initially practices these during asymptomatic periods, and once the technique is learned they are used to prevent or interrupt coughing episodes. Laryngeal irritation is often increased in chronic refractory cough. Vocal hygiene training and reducing phonotraumatic laryngeal behaviours is designed to reduce the irritation that subsequently leads to coughing. Psychoeducational counselling is used to facilitate adherence to the therapy program and address emotional issues associated with chronic refractory cough.

References

1. Blager F (ed). Cough: Increasingly seen with and without VCD. Presented at: *Advances in the Diagnosis and Treatment of Vocal Cord Dysfunction Conference*, National Jewish Medical and Research Center; 2003; Denver, Colorado.

2. Stemple J, Fry L. *Voice Therapy: Clinical Case Studies*. 3rd edn. San Diego, CA: Plural Publishing; 2009.

3. Mazzone S, McGovern AE, Cole L, Farrell MJ. Central nervous system control of cough: pharmacological implications. *Current Allergy and Asthma Reports*. 2011;11(3):265–71.

4. Davenport P. Urge to cough: What can it teach us about cough? *Lung*. 2008;186(S1):107–11.

5. Stemple J, Glaze L, Klaben B. *Clinical Voice Pathology: Theory and Management*. 4th edn. San Diego, CA: Plural Publishing; 2010.

6. Verdolini K. *Lessac–Madsen Resonant Voice Therapy: Clinician Manual*. San Diego, CA: Plural Publishing, 2008.

7. Groher M, Crary M. *Dysphagia: Clinical Management in Adults and Children*. Missouri, MO: Mosby Elsevier; 2010.

8. Graham J. Basic breathing techniques for VCD. Presented at: *Advances in the Diagnosis and Treatment of Vocal Cord Dysfunction Conference*, National Jewish Medical and Research Center; 2003; Denver, Colorado.

9. Newsham K, Klaben B, Miller V, Saunders J. Paradoxical vocal cord dysfunction: Management in athletes. *Journal of Athletic Training*. 2002;37(3):325–8.

10. Murry T, Branski R, Yu K, *et al.* Laryngeal sensory deficits in patients with chronic cough and paradoxical vocal fold movement disorder. *The Laryngoscope*. 2010;120:1576–81.

11. Mathers-Schmidt B, Brilla L. Inspiratory muscle training in exercise-induced paradoxical vocal fold motion. *Journal of Voice*. 2005;19(4):635–44.

12. Erickson-Levendoski E, Sivasankar M. Investigating the effects of caffeine on phonation. *Journal of Voice*. 2011;25(5):215–9.

13. Milner M. Desensitizing to irritants with vocal cord dysfunction. Presented at: *Advances in the Diagnosis and Treatment of Vocal Cord Dysfunction Conference*, National Jewish Medical and Research Center; 2003; Denver, Colorado.

14. Franca M. Effects of hydration on voice performance: Ph.D. Dissertation. Southern Illinois University, Carbondale; 2006.

15. Hartley NA, Thibeault SL. Systemic hydration: relating science to clinical practice in vocal health. *Journal of Voice*. 2014;28(5):652.e1–.e20.

16. Verdolini K, Titze I, Druker D. Changes in phonation threshold pressure with induced conditions of hydration. *Journal of Voice*. 1990;4:142–51.

17. Paul I, Beiler J, McMonagle A, *et al*. Effect of honey, dextromethorphan, and no treatment on nocturnal cough and sleep quality for coughing children and their parents. *Archives of Pediatric Adolescent Medicine*. 2007;161(12):1140–6.

18. Verdolini Abbott K, Li NYK, Branski R, *et al*. Vocal exercise may attenuate acute vocal fold inflammation. *Journal of Voice*. 2012;26(6):814.e1–.e13.

19. Behrman A. Facilitating behavioural change in voice therapy: The relevance of motivational interviewing. *American Journal of Speech Language Pathology*. 2006;15:215–25.

20. Wye P. Motivational Interviewing. *Motivational Interviewing Workshop*; 6/3/2013; Newcastle, Australia. 2013.

10

Personalising the treatment program for chronic refractory cough

Anne E. Vertigan

The preceding chapter provides an overview of the speech pathology treatment program for chronic refractory cough. Like most speech pathology programs, treatment needs to be adapted to needs of the individual patient. Treatment programs for chronic refractory cough should target the specific characteristics of the individual patient.

This chapter outlines the process for designing an individual treatment program. Appendix 11 provides a format to assist the speech pathologist design a treatment plan and can assist problem-solving during follow-up sessions. Although this information may be intuitive, it provides a structured method of developing a treatment program based on the individual patient's assessment results.

The following considerations are included in the therapy plan.

1. **Therapy schedule:** The therapy schedule includes an estimate of the number, length and frequency of therapy sessions.
2. **Choice of symptom suppression exercises:** These exercises may change throughout the course of treatment, depending on their effectiveness for the individual patient.
3. **Recommended implementation of symptom suppression exercises:** For example, during symptom free periods or at the first sign of cough.
4. **Therapy goals:** Examples of therapy goals include

    a. to identify precipitating sensation and substitute with strategy;

    b. to reduce laryngeal irritation;

    c. to improve symptom control;

    d. to improve voice quality; and

    e. to improve efficiency of phonation.

5. **Other recommendations:** The treatment plan might include other recommendations such as specific vocal hygiene strategies, or recommendations for further investigation.

In patients presenting with combined cough and paradoxical vocal fold movement, it may be preferable to target one symptom at a time. Targeting multiple symptoms and giving numerous exercises can be confusing and overwhelming for the patient. It is more difficult to perfect the cough suppression technique when learning multiple techniques simultaneously. Patients may present with several symptoms and the selection of the symptom to target first in therapy is variable. It often involves targeting the most significant symptom for the patient. If cough is thought to be an attempt to release paradoxical vocal fold movement, then paradoxical vocal fold movement may need to be controlled first.

Specific treatment strategies for the individual patient are outlined in the following sections and summarised in Table 10.1. This section should be regarded as a guide on which to base clinical judgement rather than a rigid prescription.

Reflux

Patients with gastroesophageal reflux disease (GERD) who have had previous anti-reflux treatment may have persisting reflux symptoms. Lifestyle strategies for reflux can be incorporated into the treatment program. These lifestyle strategies include: (1) Weight loss, (2) Raising the head of the bed, (3) Small frequent meals rather than large meals, (4) Reducing tight clothing, (5) Avoiding eating before reclining, (6) Diet modification, including reducing alcohol, spicy, acidic or fatty food, and (7) Chewing gum.[1] When raising the head of the bed, patients need to be encouraged to actually raise the bed by placing house bricks or equivalent under the legs of the head of the bed. Propping up on pillows is not sufficient. Although it is not the role of the speech pathologist to provide advice about medication, patients may need encouragement to take their prescribed medication.

Medical

    Gastroesophageal reflux disease

    Increase Reflux Symptom Index Score

    Asthma

    Respiratory disease other than asthma

Voice

    Increased voice handicap index score

    Professional voice user

    Dysphonia identified during initial
        assessment/voice screening

    Cough triggered by voice assessment
        tasks

Cough Characteristics

    Limited warning before cough

    Deliberate coughing

    Nocturnal cough

    Pattern of cough

    Cough worse after eating

    Cough Triggers

Respiratory Characteristics

    Respiratory difficulty

    Habitual breathing pattern

    Breath-holding

Emotional/psychological characteristics

    Anxiety or depression

    Patient motivation

Physical characteristics

    Oromusculature/cranial nerve charac-
        teristics

    Excess musculature tension

Table 10.1: Patient characteristics..

Asthma

Forrest[2] confirmed paradoxical vocal fold movement in 75% of patients with asthma who were referred for paradoxical vocal fold movement evaluation. Patients with combined paradoxical vocal fold movement and asthma require speech pathology intervention to distinguish between asthma and paradoxical vocal fold movement symptoms and gain voluntary control over their paradoxical vocal fold movement symptoms.

The patient will often need reassurance that they have been diagnosed with combined asthma and paradoxical vocal fold movement, especially if they believe their symptoms are solely due to asthma.

Asthma management advice is the role of the respiratory physician and respiratory nurse, however the speech pathologist may also play a role in encouraging compliance with the asthma management plan. Some patients with asthma may be referred for non-specific upper airway dysfunction but not specifically be diagnosed with paradoxical vocal fold movement or chronic refractory cough.

Where possible, the PVFM-release exercises should be timed with the asthma medication. These exercises should be performed *before* taking preventer medication with the aim of reducing laryngeal constriction which may prevent the medication from reaching its target site of effectiveness in the lower airway. Timing of *reliever* medication and PVFM-release exercises requires more multidisciplinary team consultation. Some patients are easily able to distinguish between asthma and paradoxical vocal fold movement symptoms, and are therefore able to independently select the appropriate strategy, i.e. medication verses exercises, to relieve their symptoms. Other patients have difficulty differentiating between their symptoms and may require a more personalised plan. In some cases, the individual may be advised to perform the PVFM-release exercises at the first sign of shortness of breath, and then progress to taking reliever medication if the symptoms persist. In more severe cases, patients may need to take their reliever medication first and then progress to performing the PVFM-release exercises to reduce any co-existing laryngeal tension.

Some patients with asthma require suppression of cough and throat clearing. Strategies to improve co-ordination of respiration and phonation, including the Modified Accent Method Breathing Technique, described in Chapter 9, can be particularly helpful.

There is a degree of overlap between PVFM-release exercises and breathing exercises specifically designed for asthma. Breathing dysfunction in asthma may not be specifically due to paradoxical vocal fold movement and may be due to other habitual factors. Breathing exercises for asthma include reducing the respiratory rate, promoting nasal rather than oral respiration, and abdominal breathing.[3] Once these fundamental components have been achieved, exercises can be incorporated into standing and walking and various breath-hold patterns are introduced.[3] The speech pathology assessment of the patient with combined paradoxical vocal fold movement and asthma should take particular notice of respiratory rate, breathing route, breathing focus, consistency of breathing, presence of breath-holding, stridor, and coordination of respiration and phonation. The exercises described by Thomas[3] can be adapted for these patients and incorporated into the PVFM-release breathing. These exercises (1) ensure breathing rate is not excessive, (2) ensure nasal breathing, (3) promote abdominal breathing, with focus on lower abdominal movement, (4) vary the respiratory pattern, and (5) avoid breath-holding and constriction.

Other respiratory disease

Cough control exercises may be useful in patients with other respiratory diseases such as bronchiectasis or cystic fibrosis, who need to clear their lungs regularly. Some patients can become caught in a pattern of clearing mucous too frequently and exacerbate irritation.[4] Cough suppression in these conditions could be harmful and should only occur following consultation with the physician. In these cases, the treatment program aims to: (1) Eliminate the pattern of clearing the mucus each time the sensation that mucus is accumulating occurs, (2) wait until it is easy to expectorate the mucus, and (3) set a regular number of times per day to clear mucus by using the cough. Using cough control exercises in this manner is less irritating and therefore less likely to produce more mucus. It should be noted, however, that this program has been described but not systematically evaluated.

Dysphonia

Voice abnormalities might be identified during the case history interview or clinical examination. These abnormalities might indicate the need for more formal voice assessment or additional voice therapy techniques. These techniques may include but are not limited to resonant voice therapy, vocal function exercises, release of laryngeal constriction, semi-occluded vocal tract techniques, or modified accent method breathing.

The choice of voice therapy technique will depend on the therapy goals and the underlying disorder. For example, there may be an element of muscle tension dysphonia in addition to cough and respiratory symptoms. It may be more important to address cough and respiratory symptoms before addressing voice symptoms. However, earlier introduction of voice therapy techniques may be required if the phonatory pattern is a trigger for cough.

Limited warning before the cough

Some patients report that the cough starts with no warning and that they do not experience an urge to cough. If there is no urge to cough or warning before cough episodes, the patient will be unable to implement their cough suppression technique to prevent coughing. The patient will need to increase their awareness of their laryngeal sensation. One way of increasing this awareness is to maintain a diary of laryngeal irritation. The patient is asked to rate their urge to cough every 15 minutes throughout the day, and implement the cough suppression strategy each time the urge to cough rating reaches 2 or 3 on the urge to cough scale. Initially, the ratings may need to be completed in the clinical setting with support, before being given as home practice. The diary in Appendix 12 can be adapted for the individual patient, for example by altering the time intervals. This process may facilitate greater and more frequent attention to laryngeal irritation. It will help the patient become more aware of their urge to cough, help them to prevent the cough and be proactive in reducing their laryngeal irritation.

An alternative strategy for patients who report no warning before the cough, is to use the cough suppression technique to interrupt rather than prevent the cough. The goal in this scenario is to control the severity and duration of the cough. A third strategy is to encourage the patient to focus on those coughing and throat clearing episodes that are easy to suppress and then gradually work towards controlling the more difficult episodes. Positive reinforcement may be needed for each cough episode they are able to suppress.

Deliberate coughing

Deliberate coughing is reported by a significant proportion of patients with chronic refractory cough. This deliberate coughing pattern occurs in response to the urge to cough. The aim of treatment in this situation is to reprogram the patient's response to their urge to cough and to reduce their laryngeal irritation. Strategies to address deliberate coughing include:

1. Education that the cough and throat clearing will exacerbate rather than relieve irritation, and that nothing needs to be cleared from the airway. Sipping water, sucking non-medicated lozenges and swallowing phlegm create less irritation in the long term.
2. Reassurance that they will not be harmed by avoiding coughing.
3. Increase water intake and drink water frequently throughout the day as a substitute for coughing and throat clearing.
4. Avoid laryngeal irritants as described in Chapter 9.
5. Avoid frequent throat clearing
6. Consume soothing products such as non-medicated lozenges, chewing gum, or teaspoons of honey frequently throughout the day.

Nocturnal cough

Cough is usually less frequent at night, regardless of the cause.[5] However, nocturnal cough is difficult to address as the patient does not have the opportunity to respond to their urge to cough. If the patient complains of significant nocturnal cough, medical causes may need to be reconsidered. Attention should be paid to management of reflux, particularly to ensure that the patient continues to take their prescribed anti-reflux medication. Lifestyle management of reflux is especially important.

Placing water beside the bed at night is useful for patients with nocturnal cough. Although this strategy will not prevent the cough from occurring, it can help to reduce the severity of symptoms if the patient wakens coughing or with the urge to cough. Ideally the water should be easily accessible and in a bottle with an attachment that can be used while semi-reclining in bed rather than requiring the patient to sit upright each time they wish to drink.

Nasal breathing during sleep can reduce laryngeal irritation. While it is not possible to monitor breathing while unconscious, it may be possible to encourage nasal breathing while dropping off to sleep. This strategy has been reported to be helpful by some patients.

Pattern of coughing

The cough may be intermittent or occur continuously throughout the day. The cough suppression exercises can be tailored to the pattern of coughing. If the pattern is intermittent, the patient can be taught to increase their awareness of throat irritation and implement strategies to suppress the cough at the slightest sign of irritation. If the pattern of cough is continuous, it is better to aim for a predetermined symptom-free period(s) during the day. Initially, begin with five minutes per day and gradually progress to longer periods. Alternatively, set aside a period of time per day, where the patient focuses solely on suppressing their cough.

Some patients will attempt to suppress their cough during the initial assessment session. The speech pathologist should observe and reinforce these attempts. These attempts show that the patient is trying to exert voluntary control over the cough. If the patient is predominantly throat clearing, a behaviour modification program for throat clearing, as discussed in Chapter 9, might be appropriate.

Cough worse after eating

If the cough is worse after eating, reflux strategies should be considered. Again, check the patient's compliance with prescribed anti-reflux medication. The speech pathologist may need to liaise with the referring specialist regarding optimal reflux control. In addition, lifestyle strategies for the management of reflux cannot be underestimated.

Gum chewing has been found to raise esophageal pH.[1] Anecdotally, we have had feedback that gum chewing after meals has relieved cough symptoms in patients with cough occurring after eating. We hypothesise that the chewing and swallowing action occurring during gum chewing counteracts the reflux action and helps to suppress cough.

Triggers

The patient may have noted specific triggers during the assessment. Where possible, patients can minimise exposure to identified triggers for a short period of time in order to get the symptoms under control. Once the symptoms are under control, patients can gradually increase exposure to those triggers. Long term avoidance of triggers is not recommended as it is generally difficult to avoid exposure to triggers while participating in everyday activities. Some patients are unable to identify any specific triggers. If this is the case, then it may not be necessary to invest significant time identifying triggers.

Considerations for some of the commonly identified triggers are outlined below.

1. **Talking:** Patients for whom talking is a trigger may require voice therapy techniques, such as resonant voice therapy, to reduce hyperfunction.
2. **Eating and drinking in the absence of oropharyngeal dysphagia:** These patients may have increased laryngeal hypersensitivity.
3. **Stress and anxiety:** Patients may benefit from relaxation exercises. A referral to a mental health professional should be considered.
4. **Shortness of breath:** Ensure that associated medical conditions such as asthma are well managed. Consider a diagnosis of paradoxical vocal fold movement and treat accordingly.
5. **Odours:** Gartner-Smith[6] suggests that oral breathing can eliminate the cognitive bias associated with the odour of the stimulus. In therapy, oral breathing could be used when desensitizing patients to particular odours. It will eliminate the odour, while allowing the patient to continue breathing while exposed to the source of the odour. The response of oral breathing may help to indicate the realistic response to the particular odour.[6]

6. **Cold air:** Encourage nasal breathing, reduce the time exposed to cold temperatures, or in extreme situations, place a scarf or hand over the nose and mouth for short periods during exposure.

Respiratory difficulty

Patients with paradoxical vocal fold movement associated with cough will require specific management strategies for the paradoxical vocal fold movement, such as PVFM-release breathing. Patients should practice their PVFM-release exercises until they are proficient. They should then implement the exercises at the very first sign of breathing difficulty, cough or tightness. Severe acute episodes of paradoxical vocal fold movement or cough syncope will require an emergency management plan, as described in Chapter 9.

If breathing difficulty is observed during the assessment, the speech pathologist should ensure optimal medical management, including compliance with any asthma medications. Patients with known asthma may require further medical assessment if there is an asthma exacerbation. The patient may also require evaluation for paradoxical vocal fold movement if it has not been previously diagnosed.

Habitual breathing pattern

The patient's habitual breathing pattern might be suboptimal, particularly with increased clavicular breathing. In this case, it may be necessary to work on relaxed breathing. Have the patient feel their lower abdominal muscles, as shown in Figure 9.3. Tactile cues may be more effective than verbal instruction. Invitations to notice, rather than change movement are more likely to result in long standing change. For example, *"notice whether you are breathing quickly"* is preferable to *"breathe slowly"*.

Breath-holding

If the patient is breath-holding, simply draw their attention to breath-holding at rest and during other activities when they are observed in the clinic. The speech pathologist may invite the patient to perform various activities such as picking an object up from the floor, reaching over their head, or moving from a standing to sitting position, while noticing their breathing pattern. Inviting the patient to notice their breath-holding is more effective than telling them to keep breathing. Many patients are unaware that they are holding their breath and surprised once they begin to pay attention to the pattern. Maintaining a diary of breath-holding events, such as during gardening or housework, may be helpful.

Patients might maintain a constricted laryngeal posture with lateral narrowing of the true and false vocal folds and anterior-posterior constriction of the epiglottic and arytenoid cartilages.[7] This position may be subconsciously maintained in order to anticipate airway irritation. The partially constricted posture may not be a problem at rest, but may cause effortful and inefficient respiratory patterns during physical exertion. Similarly, removing the irritant may not be sufficient to address this constricted laryngeal pattern.[7]

Although the breath-holding pattern is often habitual, some patients report that they hold their breath in attempt to suppress their cough. The patient can be invited to breathe in gently through their nose, just to the point where they feel the irritation, and to maintain the breathing cycle in a regular rhythm.

Anxiety or depression

Supportive contact with a health professional may be adequate to address emotional issues associated with the cough. There can be an improvement in aspects of anxiety and depression as cough symptoms improve. In more severe cases, however, patients may require referral to a mental health professional.

Patient motivation

Patient motivation needs to be monitored throughout the course of therapy. Patient motivation may change throughout therapy and can be influenced by the speech pathologist. Any positive steps that the patient makes towards behaviour change should be reinforced. The reasons for the perceived lack of motivation should be explored. For example, does the patient appear poorly motivated because they believe that therapy will not help them, or because they have difficulty accepting their diagnosis? Do they understand the rationale for the therapy and see how the exercises will help them? Do they understand how to implement the recommended strategies? Are they receiving conflicting advice from another health professional? Motivational interviewing might be particularly helpful in these cases.

Oromusculature or cranial nerve abnormalities

Although rare, cranial nerve abnormalities might be discovered during the clinical assessment. These might be evidence of a pre-existing problem, or an undiagnosed condition. The patient may even be coughing due to undiagnosed oropharyngeal dysphagia and aspiration. The speech pathologist must keep an open mind to the possibility of other coexisting conditions and might need to initiate referral for further investigation. The oromusculature assessment might also reveal a dry oral cavity. This should be monitored and improvement should be expected by improving hydration. Again, although rare, abnormalities on clinical swallowing assessment may require further monitoring or assessment.

Excess muscle tension

Neck and shoulder tension is common in patients with hyperfunctional voice disorders and the therapy used for these disorders is applicable in patients with chronic refractory cough. Some patients will be aware that tension is present, whereas others have little awareness. Although the speech pathologist can indicate where they are observing tension, it is more helpful to invite the patient to notice any tension. Similar to the Lessac-Madsen Resonant Voice Therapy program,[8] ask the patient to notice whether there is any tension present in various areas of the body, or whether their posture is symmetrical. For example, *"Notice whether there is any tension in your abdomen"* or *"notice whether your shoulders feel even on both sides"*.

Patients with extrinsic laryngeal muscle tension may require stretching exercises for the neck and oromusculature, release of laryngeal constriction exercises, or circumlaryngeal massage. Many patients are unaware that there is tension in their throat and it is therefore helpful to inform the patient of tension immediately, once it is noted during the clinical assessment. Stretching exercises from the Lessac-Madsen Resonant Voice Therapy program[8] are often helpful. These exercises can be prescribed as a complete set, or individual stretches specifically selected for the patient. Rhythmic breathing should be maintained when performing the stretches, as some patients have a tendency to hold their breath when performing the exercises.

Service delivery considerations

Service delivery models

Service delivery models will differ between centres and can be influenced by the policy, procedures and funding of the individual service. Typically, patients with chronic refractory cough are seen for four sessions spread over a period of two months, although some may be seen for a more intense period of therapy. Alternative service delivery models have been used and may be beneficial. However, there is limited data on the required number, frequency or length of speech pathology sessions.

Our service trialled a brief intervention for chronic refractory cough. The traditional model had used comprehensive assessment, followed by four sessions of intervention. The brief model of intervention for chronic cough involved a single, brief, 30 minute initial session with the speech pathologist, followed by a brief follow-up session one month later. Patients were seen for a short screening and brief treatment session. The brief treatment included a 15 minute PowerPoint presentation outlining the treatment program and included education about cough, the Cough Suppression Swallow technique, and strategies to promote vocal hygiene. This study included 39 patients with chronic refractory cough. At the follow-up session, 24.2% of patients reported that their cough had significantly improved and that they did not require any further therapy. Approximately half the patients demonstrated improvement, but required further speech pathology intervention. Of these, 20% reported that the cough had resolved, but required further speech pathology intervention for associated voice and respiratory problems. The remaining 15.2% of patients had limited improvement in their symptoms.

Although there was an improvement in cough symptoms, there was no improvement in voice measures with any of the patients. This data suggests that brief intervention may be a viable option for patients with mild chronic refractory cough and few associated voice or paradoxical vocal fold movement symptoms.

Group therapy is another service delivery option that has been used with success in the broader speech pathology literature. Group dynamics may be helpful in the therapeutic process. There are, however, considerable logistical issues that need to be overcome in order for group therapy to be feasible.

Follow-up appointments

The effectiveness of intervention should be monitored consistently throughout the course of speech pathology treatment. An example of the clinical decision-making process in follow-up appointments is outlined in Figure 10.1. A form for documenting follow-up appointments is included in Appendix 13.

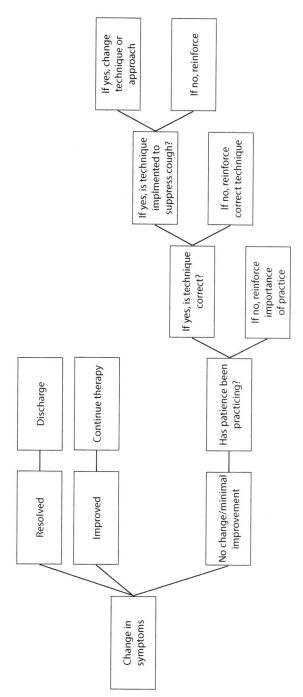

Figure 10.1: Process for managing follow-up appointments

The first issue to address during each follow-up appointment is whether or not symptoms have improved since the last appointment. At the commencement of each session, the patient is asked to estimate their degree of improvement. This estimate can be a percentage rating or visual analogue score, or alternatively, a more formal scale such as the Symptom Frequency and Severity questionnaire or Leicester Cough Questionnaire. The outcome can be classified in one of five ways: *resolved*, *improved*, *minimally improved*, *not changed*, or *deteriorated*.

If the cough has improved, the patient might simply require reinforcement of their therapy techniques and periodic review to ensure that their gains are maintained. However, if improvement has been minimal, the speech pathologist will need to investigate patient's progress more thoroughly.

If the patient reports no, or minimal change, then the first step is to determine whether or not they have been practicing their exercises. If not, then reinforce the importance of practice and problem-solve barriers to the practice. If the patient has been practicing, they can be invited to demonstrate the exercises with no cueing from the speech pathologist. This step will provide the speech pathologist with insights into how the patient is practicing at home and their ability to recall the exercises. If the technique is not performed correctly, it may require modification. Clear feedback should be given to the patient if their technique is not correct.

If the patient has been practicing and is performing the technique correctly, the next step is check whether the patient is implementing the technique at the very first sign of cough. Some patients may practice correctly but still not use the technique to inhibit their cough. Further education and problem-solving may be needed at this point. However if the patient is performing the technique correctly *and* attempting to use it to prevent their cough, then alternative therapy exercises may need to be trialled.

Previous clinical experience has shown that most patients reduce the frequency and severity of coughing and perceive better control over their cough at the conclusion of therapy, although they may still experience some residual coughing. Other patients may experience a dramatic reduction in coughing after the first treatment session. Some patients might experience improvement in cough but have persisting breathing or vocal symptoms.

Summary

Patients with chronic refractory cough present with a range of symptoms and features. Although treatment follows the same basic structure, it can be modified according to the patient's medical condition and their specific breathing, cough and voice characteristics.

References

1. Smoak B, Koufman J. Effects of gum chewing on pharyngeal and oesophageal pH. *Annals of Otology, Rhinology & Laryngology*. 2001;110(12):1117–9.

2. Forrest L, Husein T, Husein O. Paradoxical vocal cord motion: classification and treatment. *The Laryngoscope*. 2012;122:844–53.

3. Thomas M, Bruton A. Breathing exercises for asthma. *Breathe*. 2014;10(4):312–22.

4. Blager F (ed). Cough: Increasingly seen with and without VCD. Presented at: *Advances in the Diagnosis and Treatment of Vocal Cord Dysfunction Conference*, National Jewish Medical and Research Center; 2003; Denver, Colorado.

5. Birring S, Matos S, Patel R, *et al*. Cough frequency, cough sensitivity and health status in patients with chronic cough. *Respiratory Medicine*. 2006;100:1105–9.

6. Gartner-Schmidt J, Rosen C, Radhakrishnan N, Ferguson B. Odor provocation test for laryngeal hypersensitivity. *Journal of Voice*. 2006;12(3):333–8.

7. Stemple J, Fry L. *Voice Therapy: Clinical Case Studies*. 3rd edn. San Diego, CA: Plural Publishing; 2009.

8. Verdolini K. *Lessac-Madsen Resonant Voice Therapy: Clinician Manual*. San Diego, CA: Plural Publishing; 2008.

11

Speech pathology management of paradoxical vocal fold motion

Thomas Murry and Marc Haxer

Introduction

Paradoxical vocal fold motion disorder, also known as vocal cord dysfunction (VCD), is a disorder caused by episodic unintentional paradoxical adduction of the vocal folds.[1] This disorder is frequently mistaken for asthma or organic upper airway conditions[2,3] but it can also exist alongside of asthma and other pulmonary diseases.[4] PVFM presents with sudden and intense acute onset of air hunger, sense of throat constriction, stridor and dysphonia at times, elevated neck and chest muscle tension, and cough. PVFM often results in emergent medical interventions and/or prolonged trials of pharmacologic management that frequently do not result in alleviation of the presenting dyspnea. As a result, patients can experience side effects of prescribed medications along with frustration secondary to lack of progress in treating the episodes of dyspnea.[3,5] Diagnosis of PVFM is often challenging for the otolaryngologist as well as for the speech language pathologist as it may be associated with gastroesophageal reflux, stress, high level activity and even psychological aspects related to the need to acquire secondary gains.[6] However, the majority of patients appear to have treatable organic etiologies.[7] In patients with PVFM, episodic glottic obstruction may occur rapidly with or without a known trigger. The result is uncontrolled adduction of the vocal folds, primarily during the inspiratory phase of respiration and, in some instances, adduction during both the inspiratory and expiratory phases.[2,5,8–20] Although studies describing the symptomatology of PVFM began to emerge in the 1970s and 1980s, mention of a laryngeal focus to episodes of dyspnea was reported in the medical literature as early as 1842.[21,22]

The current state of the art with regard to PVFM is comparable to the ancient Hindu tale of the elephant and six blind men. Because none of the men can see the elephant as a whole, each describes the beast according to what he can feel: the elephant is a rope (tail); the elephant is a tree trunk (leg); the elephant is a wall (side of body); and so forth.[3] Even though it has been reported in the medical literature for over three decades, the existing knowledge base of this disorder remains fragmented, incomplete, and biased according to the perspective of the treating medical specialty. The lack of clarity regarding PVFM can be further attributed to the imprecise and inexact terminology used to describe this disorder by as many as 12 different medical specialties and 76 different names.[3,13]

Etiology and differential diagnosis

A number of causal factors for PVFM have been proposed. Initially, PVFM was felt to stem from increased stress and/or psychological issues.[8–11,14,15] This view remains a component of PVFM in more recent publications.[18,20,23] Laryngeal hyper reactivity or hyper responsiveness secondary to a laryngeal sensory deficit has been proposed.[12,14,16,19,23–26] Other postulated causal factors include a central neurologic focus secondary to brainstem compression, cortical or upper motor neuron injury, nuclear or lower motor neuron injury, or movement disorder and laryngeal irritation secondary to laryngopharyngeal reflux.[18] Presenting symptoms of a laryngeal respiratory dystonia that mimic those of PVFM have been described by Grillone, et al.[27] Symptoms differ from PVFM in that dyspnea associated with this condition is not episodic but persistent throughout the day. Fatigue, secondary to increased effort of breathing, may be reported. Frequently, a dystonia or tremor is present in other parts of the body. Finally, symptoms are not present when sleeping. There are also numerous other medical conditions that present with compromised respiration as a component and which need to be ruled out as causal factors in episodes of dyspnea (Table 11.1).

Evaluation and treatment

Arriving at the diagnosis of PVFM includes findings gathered from a plethora of examinations/evaluations completed by multiple medical disciplines and is often one of exclusion.[5,11,13,17,18,20] The clinical history provides clues critical

Unilateral/bilateral vocal fold motion
   impairment (abductory)

Reinke's edema

Laryngeal papilloma

Laryngeal carcinoma

Vocal Fold Granuloma

Laryngospasm

Paradoxical Vocal Fold Motion

Pertussis

Cough

Adductory Laryngeal Breathing Dystonia

Acute infection (e.g. croup, laryngitis,
   epiglottitis)

Allergies

Laryngomalacia

Tracheomalacia/Stenosis

Foreign body in airway

Extrinsic/intrinsic airway compression by
   tumor inferior to glottis

Increased neck, upper chest, shoulder
   muscle tension

Airway tumors

Table 11.1: Upper airway issues that can compromise respiration.

to generating the diagnosis of PVFM. Initial focus should be centered on the patient's perception or description of their breathing problem. When asked to identify the location of their restricted air movement, many patients will localize to the neck/laryngeal area. Some patients will initially identify the chest as the area where they feel airway restriction. Further questioning about involvement of the neck or throat area may elicit a change in the patient's focus of restricted air movement. Obtaining information relative to the patterns of restricted air movement as well as information relative to the onset of the same is also important.[18] Identification of triggers such as exertion, exposure to odors/irritants, changes in temperature or humidity, and so forth is essential in order to assist in planning proactive versus reactive behavioral management of episodes. Administration of the Reflux Symptom Index[28] yields information relative to potential irritation of the laryngeal complex secondary to refluxed stomach contents. Results of pulmonary function and laboratory findings assist in identifying the type and reason(s) for airway obstruction. With regard to potential PVFM, the flow-volume loop is the most commonly mentioned test of pulmonary function testing.[13] A flattened inspiratory loop on this evaluation suggests an extra thoracic upper airway component to dyspnea during symptomatic episodes. Completion of flexible endoscopy, either during symptomatic episodes or during completion of various provocative maneuvers such as exertion, panting, rapid deep inhalations, exposure to reported triggers, laughing, and phonation, will provide visual information relative to vocal fold function during different laryngeal functions.[10,11,18,20] Finally, results of psychological test-

185

ing assist in ruling out a psychological component to episodes of dyspnea focal to the larynx. Completion of evaluations by a number of disciplines allows for comprehensive multidisciplinary management, as well as forging close working relationships between numerous professionals throughout the diagnostic and treatment process.[13]

Behavioral intervention for the management of PVFM is focal to expanding patient knowledge of normal laryngeal respiratory function and understanding the changes that occur during the episodes. Other elements of behavioral therapy include increasing body awareness, teaching relaxed breathing, and training the patient in rescue breathing techniques for avoidance and recovery of PVFM episodes.[29] Increasing body awareness allows the patient to improve their perception of physiologic cues that suggest the imminent onset of an episode. During an episode, patients will frequently report elevated levels of upper torso muscle tension. Use of negative practice such as toggling back and forth between conscious tightening of specific muscle groups, followed by relaxation of the same, fosters greater patient awareness of the sensation of tight versus relaxed and allows for conscious decreasing of upper torso muscle tension in a controlled therapeutic setting. Once awareness of relaxed muscles is achieved in this manner, carryover of conscious relaxation into episodes can be initiated.

Given the frequent interruptions in the normal process of respiration encountered by individuals with PVFM, incoordination between inhalation and exhalation is frequently demonstrated. When this is observed by the clinician or reported by the patient, exercises designed to enhance the capture of a full breath followed by a controlled exhalation may be incorporated into therapy. Once the above strategies are habituated, training in use of breathing recovery exercises,[5,13,29,30] can be initiated. The focus of this component of intervention is to increase patient control of laryngeal respiratory function when asymptomatic. Once control is achieved in this manner, patients are encouraged to initiate use of these strategies as soon as they suspect the risk for episode onset has developed. Varying techniques have been advanced by the above authors. Mathers-Schmidt[13] suggests inhalation be accomplished with use of nasal breathing while exhaling against increased resistance using sibilant phonemes such as /s/, /ʃ/, or /f/. Coordination of breathing with increased awareness of abdominal movement is also emphasized.

Blager[30] advocates training and use of relaxed throat breathing. Emphasis is placed on learning to inhale with the tongue on the floor of the mouth, the lips

Quiet rhythmic breathing

Exhaling with shoulders relaxed, abdominal movement in/out consistent, with continuous exhalation/inhalation.

Breathing with vocal resistance

Exhaling while sustaining /ʃ/, /f/, /z/ for increasing lengths of time.

Pulsed exhalation

Produce pulse of air using /ha/ or /ʃa/ followed by sniffing in through the nose with closed mouth.

Abdominal focus at rest

Lie flat with small book on stomach, focus on elevation of book with inhalation and lowering of book with exhalation; when successful, straw breathing initiated to increase resistance while focusing on abdominal movement; exercise expanded to include sitting/standing.

Table 11.2: Protocol for respiratory retraining (Murry and Sapienza[5]).

gently closed, and the jaw gently released. Exhalation is achieved on a gentle sustained /s/, /ʃ/, or /f/. These exercises are also practiced with a focus on lower chest wall movement which allows for diverting attention away from the neck and upper chest areas during episodes. Emphasis is also placed on maintaining a pattern of repeat exhalations, as this is the easiest component of the respiratory process to maintain when symptomatic. Sandage[29] advocates use of deep nasal sniffs, which result in vocal fold abduction, followed by a slow, complete exhalation on the /s/ phoneme. The latter allows for increased air pressure at the level of the glottis, thus preventing laryngeal narrowing during exhalation. Murry and Sapienza[5] describe a program of respiratory retraining involving a sequence of exercises that move from low breathing effort to breathing against increased resistance. This protocol is contained within Table 11.2. Exercises to increase patient control of laryngeal function during episodes of PVFM should be practiced multiple times per day to increase familiarity with the same. Repeat practice sessions also contribute to an enhanced *"I can manage my breathing problem"* focus from the patient.

PVFM is a common etiology of dyspnea in athletes, both competitive and recreational. PVFM can also exist with asthma and exercise-induced breathing disorders of the upper airway such as bronchospasm. PVFM may contribute to exercise-related respiratory symptoms more frequently in middle school- and high school-aged athletes than in college athletes. Classic symptoms of stridor and/or hoarseness are often not present in athletes with PVFM, even during high energy output. Accurate diagnosis of asthma, bronchospasm and PVFM requires objective testing in order to prevent patients from being subjected to medications that are ineffective and that may have potential side effects for certain individuals. Sandage[29] suggests these individuals are often high achievers in the classroom and in sports. The goal in working with this patient population is to keep them in their games and avoid breaks in performance. As with the non-athletic patient, breathing recovery exercises are utilized to keep the throat open until the feeling of constriction passes. Once respiration is stabilized, the athlete can return to mouth breathing during exertion. Some athletes engage in breath-holding during practice and performance; additional breathing training may be needed to keep the throat open during extreme exertion. Behavioral intervention with athletes may differ dependent on their sport. With swimmers, deep nasal sniffs can work with specific training for each stroke or event. Use of the nose as a pathway for inspiration may not be possible with some swimmers. In this case, use of pulsed pursed lip inhalation may allow for greater alleviation of air hunger. Runners can practice their modified breathing strategies while on a treadmill or track at a relatively slow pace picking up their pace as use of modified breathing becomes tolerated. If episodes of PVFM are predictable, e.g., running up a hill, 15 minutes into exertion, etc., athletes should initiate use of recovery exercises prior to the increase in risk to avoid and event. It is paramount that athletes initially practice their rescue breathing outside of their sport to gain mastery over their recovery strategies. Once this is achieved, carryover of their strategies into their athletic practice/performance can be undertaken. Ruddy, et al.[32] and Mathers-Schmidt and Brilla[33] have advocated use of inspiratory muscle strength trainers. These are devices which are used to increase the strength of inspiratory muscles, thus allowing for improved respiratory function during elevated levels of exertion. Regardless of the strategy(ies) used, the goal of respiratory retraining with athletes is practicing regular and recovery breathing at various levels of exertion without experiencing air hunger.

In some cases, symptoms of laryngopharyngeal and gastroesophageal reflux may contribute to the symptoms of air hunger. Thus, proper assessment and treatment of reflux may be a necessary component of PVFM management.[18]

Treatment of reflux may only involve dietary management or can be expanded to include use of over the counter liquid antacids, H2 blockers, proton pump inhibitors, or a combination of these medications at the physician's discretion. Speech pathologists should encourage patients whose PVFM treatment regimen includes reflux management to maintain their adherence to physician-directed reflux management as consistently as possible. In the athlete with PVFM and reflux, avoidance of food/liquid within a two- or three-hour window of exertion, to allow for gastric emptying and return of the stomach to a minimal- to no-acid state, should be stressed. If oral intake within that time frame cannot be avoided, patients should be encouraged to discuss use of Gaviscon or Gaviscon Advance to 'blanket' digestive activity during periods of exertion.[34]

Summary

Paradoxical vocal fold motion presents the clinician with a challenging differential diagnosis. During episodes, inhalation is the most commonly compromised component of the respiratory cycle, although exhalation can also be affected. Multiple causal factors have been postulated, although a definitive reason for laryngeal closure during episodes of PVFM remains elusive. Treatment can be multi-modality in nature and must be tailored to the needs of the patient. Behavioral management of this disorder by speech-language pathologists has been shown to be efficacious.

References

1. Hoyle F. Vocal Cord Dysfunction. *Immunology and Allergy Clinics of North America*. 2013;33:1–32.

2. Altman KW, Mirza M, Ruiz C, Sataloff RT. Paradoxical vocal fold motion: presentation and treatment options. *Journal of Voice*. 2000;103(14):99–103.

3. Brugman SM. What's this thing called vocal cord dysfunction? Retrieved 6/24/2008 at http://chestnet.org/education/online/pccu/vol20/lessons25_27/print26.php

4. Matrka L. Paradoxic vocal fold movement disorder. *Otolaryngologic Clinics of North America*. 2014;47(1):135–46.

5. Murry T, Sapienza C. The role of voice therapy in the management of paradoxical vocal fold motion, chronic cough, and laryngospasm. *Otolaryngologic Clinics of North America*. 2010;43:73–83.

6. Maschka DA, Bauman NM, McCray PB, *et al*. A classification scheme for paradoxical vocal fold motion. *The Laryngoscope*. 1997;107:1429–35.

7. Hartnick CJ. Boseley ME. *Pediatric Voice Disorders*, 255–6. San Diego, CA: Plural Publishing; 2008.

8. Patterson R, Schatz M, Horton, M. Munchausen's stridor: non-organic laryngeal obstruction. *Clinical Allergy*. 1974;4:307–10.

9. Appleblatt, NH, Baker, SR. Functional upper airway obstruction. *Archives of Otolaryngology - Head and Neck Surgery*. 1981;107:305–6.

10. Christopher KL, Wood II RP, Eckert RC, *et al*. Vocal Cord Dysfunction Presenting as Asthma. *New England Journal of Medicine*. 1983;308:1566–70.

11. Martin RJ, Blager FL, Gay ML, Wood II RP. Paradoxic Vocal Cord Motion in Presumed Asthmatics. *Seminars in Respiratory Medicine*. 1987;8:332–7.

12. Andrianopoulos MV, Gallivan GJ, Gallivan KH. PVCM, PVCD, EPL, and irritable larynx syndrome: what are we talking about and how do we treat it? *Journal of Voice*. 2000;14:607–18.

13. Mathers-Schmidt BA. Paradoxical vocal fold motion: a tutorial on a complex disorder and the speech pathologist's role. *American Journal of Speech-Language Pathology*. 2001;10:111–25.

14. Morris MJ, Allan PF, Perkins PJ. Vocal cord dysfunction etiologies and treatment. *Clinical Pulmonary Medicine*. 2006;13(2):73–86.

15. Vertigan AE, Theodoros DG, Gibson PG, Winkworth AL. The relationship between chronic cough and paradoxical vocal fold movement: a review of the literature. *Journal of Voice*. 2006;20(3):466–80.

16. Cukier-Blaj S, Bewley A, Aviv JE, Murry T. Paradoxical vocal fold motion: a sensory-motor laryngeal disorder. *The Laryngoscope*. 2008;118:367–70.

17. Hicks M., Brugman SM, Katial R. Vocal cord dysfunction/paradoxical vocal fold motion. *Primary Care Clinics - Office Practice*. 2008;35:81–103.

18. Koufman JA, Block C: Differential diagnosis of paradoxical vocal fold movement. *American Journal of Speech-Language Pathology*. 2008;17:327–34.

19. Murry T, Branski RC, Yu K, *et al*. Laryngeal sensory deficits in patients with chronic cough and paradoxical vocal fold movement disorder. *The Laryngoscope*. 2010;120:1576–81.

20. Forrest LA, Husein T, Husein O. Paradoxical Vocal Cord Motion: Classification and Treatment. *The Laryngoscope*. 2012;122:844–53.

21. Lacy TJ, McManis SE. On vocal cord dysfunction. *Military Medicine*. 1993;158(4):A4.

22. Christopher KL, Morris MJ. Vocal cord dysfunction, paradoxic vocal fold motion, or laryngomalacia? Our understanding requires an interdisciplinary approach. *Otolaryngologic Clinics of North America*. 2010;43:43–66.

23. Balkissoon R, Kenn K. Asthma: vocal cord dysfunction (VCD) and other dysfunctional breathing disorders. *Seminars in Respiratory and Critical Care Medicine*. 2012;33:595–605.

24. Morrison M, Rammage L, Emami AJ. The irritable larynx syndrome. *Journal of Voice*. 1999;13:447–55.

25. Vertigan AE, Theodoros DG, Gibson PG, Winkworth AL. Voice and upper airway symptoms in people with chronic cough and paradoxical vocal fold movement. *Journal of Voice*. 2007;21(3):361–83.

26. Morrison M, Rammage L. The irritable larynx syndrome as a central sensitivity syndrome. *Canadian Journal of Speech-Language Pathology and Audiology*. 2010;34(4):282–9

27. Grillone GA, Blitzer A, Brin MF, *et al*. Treatment of adductor laryngeal breathing dystonia with Botulinum Toxin Type A. *The Laryngoscope*. 1994;10430–2.

28. Belafsky PC, Postma GN, Koufman JA. Validity and reliability of the Reflux Symptom Index (RSI). *Journal of Voice*. 2002;16(2):274–7.

29. Sandage M. Sniffs, gasps and cough: treatment of irritable larynx syndrome across the lifespan. Paper presented at the *Concepts in Voice Therapy Conference*, New Orleans, LA; 2009.

30. Blager FB. Symptoms and treatment of vocal cord dysfunction/paradoxical vocal fold motion. Short Course presented at the *Annual Convention of the American Speech-Language-Hearing Association*, Chicago, IL; 2008

31. Hanks CD, Parsons J, Benninger C, *et al*. Etiology of dyspnea in elite and recreational athletes. *The Physician and Sportsmedicine*. 2012(May);40(2):28–33.

32. Ruddy BH, Davenport P, Baylor J, *et al*. Inspiratory muscle strength training and behavioral therapy in a case of a rower with exercise induced paradoxical vocal fold dysfunction. *International Journal of Pediatric Otorhinolaryngology*. 2004;68(10):1327–32.

33. Mathers-Schnidt BA, Brilla LR. Inspiratory muscle training in exercise-induced paradoxical vocal fold motion. *Journal of Voice*. 2005;19(4):635–44.

34. Phyland D. Therapy for the misbehaving larynx – VCD, ILS, and cough. Paper presented at the *13th Biennial Phonosurgery Symposium Workshops*, Madison, WI; 2014.

12

Speech pathology management of globus pharyngeus

Anne E. Vertigan and Peter G. Gibson

The treatment of globus pharyngeus is relevant to the discussion of chronic cough and paradoxical vocal fold movement as many patients present to their doctor or speech pathologist with overlapping symptomatology. The description of treatment for globus pharyngeus in this chapter has been included to assist the clinician manage patients presenting with either globus pharyngeus in isolation, or in combination with cough and paradoxical vocal fold movement.

Symptoms in globus pharyngeus

The term *globus* is derived from the Latin word for *ball* and means a sensation of a lump or foreign body in the throat.[1,2] It occurs in the absence of oropharyngeal dysphagia but, nevertheless, can be quite distressing for the individual. The symptoms are often relieved during swallowing.[3] Salleslagh, *et al.*[4] describe globus pharyngeus as a one of several functional gastrointestinal disorders. It is more prevalent in middle age, accounting for 3–4% of referrals to otolaryngologists.[5] True idiopathic globus should be differentiated from globus occurring in the presence of a structural lesion, for example vocal fold polyp, or cervical osteophyte.[4] Globus pharyngeus can co-occur with other functional gastrointestinal disorders such as irritable bowel syndrome. This co-occurrence might suggest underlying visceral hypersensitivity.[4]

Globus pharyngeus is a benign, non-progressive condition.[6] Classic symptoms of globus pharyngeus are a sensation of a lump in the throat[7] and may also include food sticking when swallowing, persistent need to swallow, excess saliva and phlegm.[5] The specific location of symptoms is variable and is often not specified in studies of the condition.[4]

Globus pharyngeus occurs in the absence of dysphagia[4] and symptoms may be less severe when eating.[2] Of patients with globus pharyngeus, 70% have no swallowing problems.[2]

A recent study compared symptoms and quantitative sensory testing in patients with a range of laryngeal conditions including globus pharyngeus, chronic refractory cough, and paradoxical vocal fold movement.[8] Laryngeal sensation in patients with globus pharyngeus was abnormal compared to healthy controls, but not significantly different from patients with other laryngeal conditions. Symptoms of breathing difficulty, voice and upper airway irritation were also higher in patients with globus pharyngeus than healthy controls. The mean Timed Swallow Test result was $17\,ml/sec$ $(SD = 12)$, which is within the normal range.[8] However, this result was significantly lower than healthy controls and similar to the patients with chronic refractory cough, paradoxical vocal fold movement and muscle tension dysphonia. Cough reflex sensitivity and cough frequency (coughs per hour) were increased, compared to healthy controls, but better than patients in the other clinical groups. Voice measures, including the Voice Handicap Index, auditory perceptual voice ratings and maximum phonation times, were more impaired in patients with globus pharyngeus than healthy controls, and similar to patients with chronic refractory cough and paradoxical vocal fold movement.[8]

As expected, however, voice measures were less severe in the patients with globus pharyngeus than those with muscle tension dysphonia. The authors concluded that globus pharyngeus might be part of a group of laryngeal disorders with common sensory dysfunction supporting the *laryngeal hypersensitivity* hypothesis.

Etiology of globus pharyngeus

The etiology of globus pharyngeus has not been clearly defined in the literature. It is multifactorial and can be variable between patients. The etiology can include a range of medical conditions such as, enlarged tonsils, chronic sinusitis and pharyngitis,[1] and is similar to other laryngeal conditions such as chronic refractory cough and paradoxical vocal fold movement.

Irritation of the pharyngeal mucosa can also contribute to globus sensation. This irritation can be caused by laryngopharyngeal reflux though direct stimulation, referred from the lower esophageal sphincter, or hypertonicity of the upper esophageal sphincter.

A range of gastrointestinal disorders such as gastroesophageal reflux disease have been suggested in the etiology of globus pharyngeus. There is a temporal association between globus symptoms and reflux when tested with impedance manometry,[9] however no direct cause has been identified. Chen[10] examined 23 patients with globus pharyngeus. None of these patients had abnormal acid reflux, leading the authors to conclude that reflux has a limited role in the development of globus symptoms. Zelenik reported the results of pH monitoring in confirmed globus patients.[11] Reflux was present in 23.9% of patients when the pH probe was 4.0, and an additional 8.7% when the pH probe was 5.0. These results suggest that weakly acid reflux might play a role in globus pharyngeus.

Other gastrointestinal diseases occurring in globus pharyngeus include pharyngeal dysmotility, abnormal upper esophageal sphincter function and esophageal motor disorders.[1] Anatomical abnormalities associated with globus pharyngeus may include hypertrophy of the base of tongue, retroverted epiglottis, cervical heterotopic gastric mucosa,[1] osteophytes,[12,13] Zenker's diverticulum,[13] and esophageal abnormality, such as web, hiatus hernia and achalasia. More sinister etiologies may include malignancy in the laryngopharyngeal region or esophagus,[1] however malignancy rarely presents with globus sensation alone.[14] Globus can be iatrogenic following head and neck surgical procedures.[4] It can co-occur with vocal fold palsy and paradoxical vocal fold movement.[4]

Globus pharyngeus has been associated with reduced Xerostomia, which is a dry mouth caused by reduced saliva flow. Saliva is essential for maintaining the health of the oral cavity.[7] Xerostomia leads to reduced antimicrobial activity which is essential for averting the colonization of oral and pharyngeal mucosa by potential pathological organisms.[7] There is also loss of lubricating function of saliva which makes the oral and pharyngeal cavities more vulnerable to physical and chemical insults.[7]

Globus symptoms have been reported in patients with thyroid disease. Burns[15] conducted a two year prospective study of 200 patients with thyroid disease and voice disorders. Fifty-eight of these patients reported globus sensation preoperatively, and 80% of these resolved postoperatively. There was no significant difference in thyroid weight and globus Visual Analogue Scale score, and no difference in globus symptoms between patients with partial and total thyroidectomy.

Psychological conditions including stress and anxiety have also been suggested in the etiology of globus pharyngeus. Anxiety may lead to increased laryngeal muscle tension which subsequently reduces the strength of the normal swallow. There can be increased somatic distress along with anxiety and depression.[2] In fact, anxiety levels along with throat symptoms are two independent predictors of the patient's reaction to their throat symptoms.[2]

The range of etiologies reported in the literature raises the question of whether globus pharyngeus is a symptom of underlying disease, or whether it is a condition in its own right. Reduced sensation and overlap with other laryngeal conditions suggests that globus pharyngeus could be part of the laryngeal sensory hyperresponsiveness syndrome.

Medical management of globus pharyngeus

The first step in the medical management of globus pharyngeus involves a detailed clinical case history followed by external examination of the head and neck,[14] including nasendoscopy.[1] Abnormal findings on laryngoscopy require further investigation and follow-up. The aim of medical management is to rule out sinister pathology, identify and treat associated diseases and to reassure the patient.[1,14] Red flags suggesting sinister pathology include dysphagia, aspiration, regurgitation, weight loss, dysphonia and pain. The clinician should also probe for overt signs of gastroesophageal reflux disease or laryngopharyngeal reflux.

Proton pump inhibitors may be used if the patient exhibits overt signs of reflux[9] however results of studies of proton pump inhibitors in globus pharyngeus are variable.[14] Lee[1] outlined an algorithm for the management of globus. Patients with a suspicion of gastroesophageal reflux disease should receive empirical treatment with a high dose proton pump inhibitor. The proton pump inhibitor dose should be titrated if symptoms have improved after three months, and should be increased if symptoms have not improved. However, if symptoms have remained unresponsive more definitive assessment may be required, including pH monitoring, endoscopy, manometry, barium swallow or videofloroscopy. More aggressive reflux treatment may be required if pathological reflux is identified following these examinations. If pathological reflux is not identified, then behavioural treatments including speech pathology, antidepressants or cognitive behavioural therapy may be considered.

The clinical utility of barium swallow and videofluoroscopic swallow study for globus pharyngeus is inconsistent in the literature. Barium swallow examinations may detect structural esophageal abnormalities that could contribute to the globus symptoms. Other findings include an abnormal curled epiglottis, and contracted base of tongue. Alaani[16] conducted an audit of 1,154 patients who had a barium swallowing examination requested for investigation of globus pharyngeus. Two thirds of the examinations were completely normal. Less than 20% of patients had reflux, however not all had evidence of gastroesophageal reflux disease, while 15% had benign pathologies such as cervical osteophytes. Only 1% of cases (12 patients) had suspicious pathologies, none of which showed malignancy on further pharyngo-esophagoscopy. The authors suggested that barium swallow examinations should not be requested systematically as part of management of globus pharyngeus. Other authors report that barium swallows are insensitive and may even fail to detect malignancies.[9] Abnormalities may be present on barium swallow, however it is unknown whether these are more prevalent than in the general population and whether there is a causal relationship between these findings and the globus symptoms.

A Videofluoroscopic Swallow Study, also known as a Modified Barium Swallow, might also be recommended in the investigation of globus pharyngeus. Chen[12] reported the results of videofluoroscopy in 23 patients with globus pharyngeus who had no abnormalities on otolaryngology examination. All patients had normal esophageal function. Cervical osteophytes were present in ten patients. Eight patients had an abnormal pharyngeal function characterised by aspiration,[5] valleculae and piriform fossa pooling,[2] and poor laryngeal elevation.[2] It is unclear whether these abnormalities were the cause of symptoms in these patients. Prospective studies comparing videofluoroscopic swallow studies between patients with globus pharyngeus and healthy controls would be necessary to determine the clinical significance of these findings.

Although reassurance is often suggested and successful, it may be insufficient for many patients, particularly if there is associated anxiety.[14] These patients may require more extensive cognitive behavioural therapy, or speech pathology intervention. Speech pathology treatment may be particularly important if there are phonotraumatic behaviours, such as throat clearing.[14]

Cheng et al.[17] reported treatment outcomes of 30 patients with globus pharyngeus who underwent transnasalesophagoscopy. Neoplasm was excluded in all patients. The transnasalesophagectomy was followed by two weeks of proton pump inhibitor medication and written educational material regarding lifestyle modification. These modifications included vocal rest, reducing stress, reducing smoking, eliminating alcohol, treatment of underlying allergy, eliminating snoring, treating gastroesophageal reflux disease, increasing humidity and increasing fluid intake. The authors reported improved subjective symptoms and erythema of arytenoids, and reduced vocal fold oedema following treatment.

Speech pathology assessment of globus pharyngeus

The speech pathology assessment of the patient with globus pharyngeus will depend on the reason for referral and the previous tests that have occurred. Patients may be referred to speech pathology with a pre-existing diagnosis of globus pharyngeus, following nasendoscopy. Alternatively, patients may be referred to speech pathology for clinical management of a related condition, such as chronic refractory cough, paradoxical vocal fold movement, or dysphagia, and yet the speech pathologist suspects globus pharyngeus based on their assessment. The assessment of globus pharyngeus has some similarity to the assessment of chronic refractory cough and paradoxical vocal fold movement.

The case history interview should encompass the onset, duration and characteristics of the symptoms, associated medical conditions and treatment, and social history. Vocal hygiene and hydration should be considered as outlined in Chapter 8. If these issues are suboptimal they may need to be addressed during the treatment program as outlined in Chapter 9. The case history interview is an excellent opportunity for the speech pathologist to investigate the patient's understanding, concerns and beliefs regarding their condition. Some patients are concerned that they are choking, or that their symptoms are the result of serious medical disease. Some are fearful that the doctor has missed a critical finding during the medical examination.

Symptom self-rating tools provide a comprehensive profile of the nature and severity of symptoms. The Glasgow Edinburgh Throat Scale (GETS)[2,18] has been specifically designed for patients with globus pharyngeus. The GETS identifies similar symptom clusters to the Reflux Symptom Index. It contains 12 items related to throat discomfort, which are rated on an eight point scale ranging from 0 *none*, or *not at all*, to 8 *unbearable*, *extensive*, or *all the time*. Examples include *feeling something stuck*, *want to swallow all the time*, and *throat discomfort or irritation*. The Laryngeal Hypersensitivity Questionnaire, described in Chapter 8, helps understand the patient's perception of laryngeal discomfort.

The John Hunter Hospital Symptom Frequency and Severity Questionnaire and Reflux Symptom Index, also described in Chapter 8 can be useful tools and help monitor changes following therapy.

Clinical assessment will be influenced by the specific symptoms reported by the patient and the reason for the referral. If the patient has been referred for dysphagia, or has complaints regarding swallowing then a clinical swallowing assessment including assessment of oromusculature, cranial nerves, airway protection and swallowing trials[3] should be administered. During this assessment, the speech pathologist should be alert for signs of anxiety surrounding eating. The size of the bolus taken by the patient during swallowing trials can be revealing. Some patients with globus symptoms spontaneously consume enormous bolus sizes and symptoms decrease once they reduce the bolus size. Other patients may take excessively small bolus sizes. This may be due to anxiety regarding eating or previous experience of swallowing difficulty. The Timed Swallow Test[19] can provide an objective measure of swallow efficiency and bolus size. Explanation of the clinical swallowing assessment results can reassure patients that their results are falling within the normal range.

Clinical observations related to laryngeal function include the presence of cough and throat clearing during the session, and activities that exacerbate throat clearing and tension in the shoulders, upper chest and extrinsic laryngeal area. Some tension may only become evident on physical palpation. Observation of breathing might reveal information about laryngeal tension and irritation. Does the patient use a clavicular or diaphragmatic pattern? Is breathing relaxed or rapid and shallow? Does the patient have a tendency to breath hold? Patients presenting with coexisting signs of dysphonia may require further voice assessment.

Speech pathology treatment of globus pharyngeus

Several studies have reported successful outcomes from speech pathology intervention for patients with globus pharyngeus. Millicahp[5] described a treatment program for 14 patients with globus using a pre-post-test design. In this program, patients had the GETS and video fluoroscopic swallow study performed at pre-treatment. Treatment included an explanation of globus, including swallow physiology and abnormal features of swallow function. Education included the role of the tongue in propelling the bolus posteriorly and creating sufficient pressure above the upper esophageal sphincter, and the consequences of reduced laryngeal excursion to open upper esophageal sphincter and bolus transit. The patient's specific symptoms were explained and their own video fluoroscopic swallow studies were shown. Home practice included increasing the taste, temperature and texture of food, effortful swallow to increase the pressure generated by tongue base on the bolus as it passes through upper esophageal sphincter, and the Mendelsohn technique. The exercises were to be performed five times a day. Post treatment results eight weeks later showed a significant improvement in the GETS but no physiological improvement in video fluoroscopic swallow studies.

Khalil[20] conducted a randomised trial comparing speech pathology exercises (SPE) with reassurance by a nurse practitioner (RNP). In this study, forty patients were randomised to receive either SPE or RNP. Symptom scores were measured on a visual analogue scale at baseline and three months following intervention. SPE involved explanation of globus pharyngeus including the role of stress in exacerbating symptoms, reassurance that it is a benign disorder, elimination of throat clearing, adequate hydration, reducing irritating substances and finally exercises to relieve pharyngeal and laryngeal tension such as yawn, giggle posture and wet swallow rather than dry swallow. Patients were requested to repeat the exercises at home on a daily basis. RNP involved providing verbal information about globus pharyngeus and reassurance. Both sessions involved a single visit. There was significant pre-post treatment improvement in symptom scores in the SPE group ($p=0.001$) compared to no significant change in the RNP group ($p=0.58$).

Although there is a need for further research into the treatment of globus pharyngeus, the evidence to date suggests that speech pathology intervention may be effective in treating symptoms of the condition. The following treatment program is based on previous research and our own clinical experience. The program includes education and reassurance, vocal hygiene training, swallowing exercises, relaxation and stress management and elimination of phonotraumatic behaviours. The speech pathologist can select the components relevant to the individual patient. It may not be necessary to provide each of these components to all patients.

Education and reassurance

The first stage in treatment involves education and reassurance that the patient's swallow reflex is normal and that the symptoms appear to be due to laryngeal hypersensitivity. The manner in which the education is provided can influence the patient's acceptance of the information their adherence to treatment. It is often more helpful to convey the message that *"There is a problem with your laryngeal sensation"*, rather than *"There is nothing wrong"*. Likewise, positive phrasing is helpful when describing the patient's swallow. For example, *"Your swallow reflex is well coordinated"*, is more positive than *"I can't find anything wrong with your swallow"*. The speech pathologist may explain that there are numerous nerves in the laryngeal region and therefore a small amount of stimulation can be perceived by the brain as quite significant. Reassurance that symptoms can change with therapy may reduce symptom severity, motivate the patient towards successful resolution of their symptoms[21] and improve their self-efficacy.

Vocal hygiene training

The aim of vocal hygiene training in patients with globus pharyngeus is to reduce laryngeal discomfort. Key vocal hygiene strategies include ensuring adequate hydration particularly the volume and frequency water intake, steam inhalation and avoiding irritants such as alcohol, smoke and caffeine. Vocal hygiene training should be adapted for the individual patient. If few vocal hygiene issues are identified during the initial assessment, then vocal hygiene may not require significant emphasis during the treatment. Vocal hygiene strategies described in Chapter 9 can be modified for patients with globus pharyngeus.

Swallowing

Although patients with globus pharyngeus generally have a normal swallow, dysphagia treatment exercises can be helpful in the treatment program. These exercises include safe swallow strategies, effortful swallow and saliva management. Safe swallow strategies such as sitting upright when eating and ensuring each mouthful of food is swallowed before taking another, can be helpful for patients who express or demonstrate anxiety about eating. Some patients have a fear of choking or a perception of swallowing difficulty in the absence of dysphagia. Safe swallow strategies can increase the patient's sense of control over their swallow. A chin down posture might provide a greater sense of control of the bolus in the oral cavity.

The effortful swallow technique is useful for those patients who report feeling a lump in their throat after eating. It is hypothesised that trivial quantities of pharyngeal or valleculae residue are perceived by the patient as severe and that the effortful swallow technique reduces this residue. However prospective studies would be needed to confirm this theory. Groher[3] describes the effortful swallow as swallowing with deliberate force applied to the bolus by the structures used in swallowing. The effortful swallow technique results in increased surface electromyography amplitude in submental muscles, increased pharyngeal manometric pressures due to contraction of pharyngeal constrictor muscles and increased duration of pressure in the upper pharynx.[22] An explanation of the physiological basis behind the effortful swallow technique helps facilitate the patient's understanding of the rationale for therapy.

Saliva management strategies for globus pharyngeus[7] include increasing water intake to ten cups per day, humidification, massage of saliva glands, sour juice, sugarless gum, gargling chlorhexadine and nasal saline spray three to four times a day. Baek[7] found that 60 per cent of their patients with globus pharyngeus had saliva hypofunction measured by salivary scintigraphy, and that globus severity decreased following conservative saliva management.

Relaxation and stress management

Relaxation techniques may reduce associated anxiety and tension and promote less effortful breathing. Neck and shoulder stretches may reduce excessive tension in extrinsic laryngeal muscles and promote symmetry of neck, head and shoulders with a healthy posture. Counselling, stress management, referral to mental health professionals and cognitive behavioural therapy may be needed in some situations.[1]

Eliminate phonotraumatic behaviours

Throat clearing should be eliminated if present. Throat clearing aggravates abnormal laryngeal sensation and may contribute to the perpetuation of globus symptoms. The cycle of constant throat clearing may exacerbate laryngeal discomfort.[2] The throat clearing program described in Chapter 9 can be used for patients with globus pharyngeus.

Regular swallowing and yawning can ease laryngeal discomfort. The swallow can release excessive tension of pharyngeal constrictor muscles. The yawn lowers the larynx and expands the pharynx thereby reducing excessive muscle tension in the vocal tract.[23]

Diaphragmatic breathing may be promote relaxation, and divert focus of tension from throat to the diaphragm and abdomen. This breathing pattern should emphasise a relaxed breathing pattern rather than deep breathing.

Voice exercises are indicated if there is significant associated dysphonia or if dysphonia persists following successful resolution of the globus symptoms.

Behavioural treatment for globus is usually complete within two to three sessions. If behavioural management is not successful after one month a video fluoroscopic swallow study should be considered.

Summary

Globus pharyngeus is typically considered a separate condition to chronic refractory cough and paradoxical vocal fold movement however there is some overlap between the etiology, symptoms and management of the conditions. This chapter provides an outline for a speech pathology management plan for globus pharyngeus. There is a need for more systematic research into the etiology, assessment and treatment of patients with globus pharyngeus in order to examine treatment efficacy and identify the underlying mechanism.

References

1. Lee B, Kim G. Globus pharyngeus: A review of its etiology, diagnosis and treatment. *World Journal of Gastroenterology*. 2012;18(20):2462–71.

2. Deary IJ, Wilson JA, Harris MB, Macdougall G. Globus pharyngis: Development of a symptom assessment scale. *Journal of Psychosomatic Research*. 1995;39(2):203–13.

3. Groher M, Crary M. *Dysphagia: Clinical Management in Adults and Children*. Missouri, MO: Mosby Elsevier; 2010.

4. Selleslagh M, van Oudenhove L, Pauwels A, *et al.* The complexity of globus: a multidisciplinary perspective. *Nature Reviews: Gastroenterology & Hepatology*. 2013;11:220–33.

5. Millichap F, Lee M, Pring T. A lump in the throat: Should speech and language therapists treat globus pharyngeus? *Disability & Rehabilitation*. 2004;27(3):124–30.

6. Burns P, O'Neill JP. The diagnosis and management of globus: a perspective from Ireland. *Current Opinion in Otolaryngology & Head & Neck Surgery*. 2008;16(6):503–6.

7. Baek C, Chung M, Choi J, *et al.* Role of salivary function in patients with globus pharyngeus. *Head & Neck*. 2014;32(2):244–52.

8. Vertigan A, Bone S, Gibson PG. Laryngeal sensory dysfunction in laryngeal hypersensitivity syndrome. *Respirology*. 2013;18(6):948–56.

9.   Kortequee S, Karkos PD, Atkinson H, *et al*. Management of globus pharyngeus. *International Journal of Otolaryngology*. 2013;2013:5.

10. Chen C-L, Tsai C-C, Chou AS-B, Chiou J-H. Utility of ambulatory pH monitoring and videofluoroscopy for the evaluation of patients with globus pharyngeus. *Dysphagia*. 2007;22(1):16–9.

11. Zelenik K, Matousek P, Urban O, *et al*. Globus pharyngeus and extraesophageal reflux: simultaneous pH <4.0 and pH <5.0 analysis. *The Laryngoscope*. 2010;120(11):2160–4.

12. Chen C-L, Tsai C-C, Chou AS-B, Chiou J-H. Utility of ambulatory pH monitoring and videofluoroscopy for the evaluation of patients with globus pharyngus. *Dysphagia*. 2007;22:16–9.

13. Caylakli F, Yavuz H, Erkan A, *et al*. Evaluation of patients with globus pharyngeus with barium swallow pharyngoesophagography. *The Laryngoscope*. 2006;116(1):37–9.

14. Burns P, O'Neill J. The diagnosis and management of globus: a perspective from Ireland. *Current Opinion in Otolaryngology & Head & Neck Surgery*. 2008;16(6):503–6.

15. Burns P, Timon C. Thyroid pathology and the globus symptom: are they related? A two year prospective trial. *Journal of Laryngology & Otology*. 2007;121(3):242–5.

16. Alaani A, Vengala S, Johnston MN. The role of barium swallow in the management of the globus pharyngeus. *European Archives of Oto-Rhino-Laryngology*. 2007;264(9):1095–7.

17. Cheng C-C, Fang T-J, Lee T-J, *et al*. Role of flexible transnasal esophagoscopy and patient education in the management of globus pharyngeus. *Journal of the Formosan Medical Association*. 2012;111(3):171–5.

18. Cathcart RA, Steen N, Natesh BG, *et al*. Non-voice-related throat symptoms: comparative analysis of laryngopharyngeal reflux and globus pharyngeus scales. Journal of Laryngology & Otology. 2011;125(1):59–64.

19. Nathadwarawala K, Nicklin J, Wiles C. A timed test of swallowing capacity for neurological patients. *Journal of Neurology, Neurosurgery & Psychiatry*. 1992;55(9):822–55.

20. Khalil HS, Bridger MW, Hilton-Pierce M, Vincent J. The use of speech therapy in the treatment of globus pharyngeus patients. A randomised controlled trial. *Revue de laryngologie otologie rhinologie*. 2003;124(3):187–90.

21. Wareing M, Elias A, Mitchell D. Management of globus sensation by the speech therapist. *Logopedics Phoniatrics Vocology*. 1997;22(1):39–42.

22. Daniels SK, Huckabee M-L. *Dysphagia Following Stroke*. San Diego, CA: Plural Publishing; 2008.

23. Boone D, McFarlane S, Von Berg S, Zraick R. *The Voice and Voice Therapy*. Sydney: Allyn & Bacon; 2009.

13

Evidence for behavioural management of chronic refractory cough

Anne E. Vertigan and Peter G. Gibson

The previous chapters have outlined the medical and speech pathology management of chronic cough. The current chapter discusses the efficacy of speech pathology management of chronic refractory cough and explores the mechanisms behind improvement in cough following treatment. The aim of this chapter is to inform the speech pathologist about the evidence base for the treatment and provide a clear understanding of the rationale for therapy.

Efficacy of speech pathology management of chronic refractory cough

Early outcome studies of behavioural intervention for chronic refractory cough and paradoxical vocal fold movement involved single case studies, or case series. One of the first reports of speech pathology management of chronic cough was by Gay et al.[1] who utilised a treatment program involving speech therapy, relaxation and psychotherapy in four patients with psychogenic habit cough. A critical component of the treatment program was redefinition of the illness to encourage patients to relinquish the notion of an organic cause for their symptoms. The patients who accepted their diagnosis, demonstrated reduced hospitalisation, reduced steroid use and improvements in socialisation and happiness. One patient did not accept the chronic cough diagnosis and required rehospitalisation for the cough and respiratory symptoms. Gay et al. claimed that the medical personnel should emphasise that behavioural approaches, such as those used by speech pathologists, are specific treatments for chronic cough, otherwise patients will feel unconvinced and subsequently repeatedly seek further medications.

Blager *et al.*[2] reported a similar treatment program and applied techniques such as diaphragmatic breathing, laryngeal tension reduction and psychotherapy in four patients with chronic habit cough. Two patients were fully compliant with all aspects of the program, while the other two completed the psychotherapy component without the full speech-langauge pathology component. Following treatment, all patients experienced a reduction in the severity of their coughing attacks and were able to cease taking steroid medication. However, the frequency of coughing remained unchanged in the two patients who had not completed the full speech pathology program.

Another report[3] described a treatment program for behavioural management of twelve patients with chronic cough. The program involved behaviour modification, cognitive adjustment, vocal hygiene and promoting efficiency of voicing. Results showed improvement in the ability of most patients to control their cough. There was, however, a large attrition rate with only half the patients completing the program.

Murry[4] reported on a case series of five patients with laryngopharyngeal reflux, chronic cough and paradoxical vocal fold movement. Treatment consisted of twice-daily reflux treatment with proton pump inhibitors, H2-antagonist and lifestyle modifications. In addition to the reflux treatment, patients received four respiratory training sessions with the speech pathologist over a three month period. Therapy involved breathing exercises, focusing on breathing with minimal expiratory force and with a regular rhythm. The mean self-rated cough severity reduced from 9.2 at pre-treatment to 1.3 post treatment. Reflux Symptom Index scores improved following treatment, which suggests successful treatment of reflux. The reflux medication was tapered to once-daily therapy approximately eight months later. There was an improvement in obstruction on pulmonary function testing and an improvement in the ratio of forced inspiratory vital capacity in first 0.5 seconds to the entire forced inspiratory vital capacity, i.e. from 0.58 to 0.94. This study provided a significant contribution to the current knowledge base on behavioural management of chronic refractory cough and paradoxical vocal fold movement. It also demonstrated that maximal medical treatment for reflux might improve reflux symptoms without having a significant impact on the cough.

In a subsequent study, Murry[5] reported improvement in laryngeal sensitivity and symptoms of chronic cough and paradoxical vocal fold movement following speech pathology intervention. Sixteen patients received treatment, including twice daily proton pump inhibitors and speech pathology intervention involving *respiratory retraining*. There was no significant change in overall Reflux Symptom Index scores following treatment. Paradoxical vocal fold movement resolved in 75% of patients and improved in a further 19%. Sensation improved in 94% of patients with complete resolution in 88%. Cough, throat clearing and hoarseness symptoms all improved following treatment.

Murry[5] concluded that cough associated with paradoxical vocal fold movement was due to reduced mechanosensitivity as a result of receptors being buried in the oedematous mucosa of the pharynx and larynx. Proton Pump Inhibitor treatment reduces the oedema, but patients still require therapy for behavioural component of their cough. Chronic acid irritation results in reduced mechanical sensitivity, which leads to an increased collection of particulate or irritant matter in the larynx and pharynx. The chronic cough reflex may be an adaptive mechanism which becomes habitual to clear the pharynx. Chronic cough is associated with abnormal laryngeal sensation caused by laryngopharyngeal reflux. Paradoxical vocal fold movement may occur to protect the airway from further acid exposure. Speech pathology intervention improves respiratory and phonatory characteristics, but also improves sensory response.

Another study used a single blind randomised placebo controlled design to evaluate the efficacy of speech pathology intervention for chronic refractory cough.[6] Participants with chronic cough were randomised to receive either four sessions of speech pathology intervention for cough (treatment), or an equivalent course of healthy lifestyle education (placebo). Participants in the treatment group demonstrated significantly greater improvement in symptom ratings compared to the placebo group and a significantly higher prevalence of successful outcome, based on clinical judgement. Participants in the treatment group also demonstrated a significant improvement in auditory perceptual ratings of vocal quality compared to those receiving the placebo intervention.[6] The treatment group demonstrated a significant improvement in maximum phonation time, jitter, harmonic to noise ratio, and phonation range, however the degree of change was not significantly different between the groups. This study provides level 1 evidence for the efficacy of speech pathology intervention.

Mechanisms of speech pathology treatment for chronic cough

The pathophysiology behind speech pathology treatment of chronic refractory cough is not fully understood. A number of potential concepts have been proposed, including a reduction in coexisting paradoxical vocal fold movement, improved voluntary control over the cough, placebo effect, reduced cough reflex sensitivity, behaviour modification, reduced laryngeal irritation, and improved efficiency of phonation.

The cough reflex consists of an afferent pathway, an efferent pathway and a central pathway.[7] Stimulation of mechanical or pressure cough receptors at any place along the airway can produce a cough.[8] Chung[7] argued that central sensitization of the cough may occur through integration of sensory nerves within the central nervous system to initiate exaggerated reflexes and sensations. The cough reflex is plastic rather than static, can sensitise in response to stimuli, particularly if associated with inflammation, and can be modified at any point along the pathway. It is hypothesised that the act of coughing further stimulates afferent nerves and triggers coughing. Speech pathology intervention seeks to modify both the afferent and efferent pathways of the cough reflex by reducing stimulation of the cough receptors and increasing voluntary inhibition of the cough.

Improved cough reflex sensitivity

Increased cough reflex sensitivity in chronic cough results in a lower threshold for cough, making it more susceptible to stimulation and increasing the frequency and severity of cough episodes. Voluntary cough suppression employed during speech pathology intervention may raise the threshold for cough, thereby reducing cough reflex sensitivity. Smith et al.[9] compared cough reflex sensitivity and ratings of the urge to cough amongst healthy volunteers assigned to either a psychological exercise group, a cough suppression group, whereby they were advised *to try not to cough*, or a no intervention control group. The cough threshold was significantly reduced in the psychological exercise and cough suppression groups, with no significant difference in ratings of the urge to cough between the groups. The authors concluded that psychological factors could influence cough reflex sensitivity and that reducing concern and active suppression of the cough could raise the cough threshold.

These results are consistent with Ryan et al,[10] whereby cough reflex sensitivity decreased following speech pathology intervention. In order to explore the underlying physiology behind improvement following speech pathology intervention, Ryan *et al* compared cough reflex sensitivity before and after speech pathology intervention for chronic refractory cough.[10] In this study, 24 patients with chronic refractory cough had cough reflex sensitivity assessed using capsaicin cough sensitivity testing, ambulatory cough monitoring and self-ratings of cough before speech pathology intervention, and following each session of speech pathology intervention. Results showed a significant improvement in C5 (the concentration of capsaicin required to elicit five or more coughs) and cough threshold (the concentration of capsaicin required to elicit a single cough), which indicates that the cough reflex became less sensitive. There was also a reduction in cough frequency as measured by an ambulatory cough monitor, and urge to cough ratings. These results show that speech pathology intervention for cough results in improvement in cough-related quality of life, cough frequency and cough reflex sensitivity.

Voluntary control of cough

The relationship between voluntary control of cough and reflex mechanisms underlying cough are relevant in the behavioural management of chronic refractory cough.[1,2,11] Speech pathology intervention improves the individual's capacity to voluntarily control cough, a function that is mediated by both voluntary and reflexive pathways. The role of the cerebral cortex in modulating cough is becoming increasingly understood. Speech pathology intervention is based on the assumption that individuals have the potential to exert some voluntary control over their cough. Individuals with chronic refractory cough have strong reflexive cough control and, although there is neural capacity for voluntary control, it exerts less control over the coughing mechanism.[12] It is hypothesised that the pathway for voluntary cough control is strengthened following speech pathology intervention.

The mechanisms behind voluntary control of cough in viral illness have been also investigated. Hutchings *et al.*[13] examined voluntary suppression of cough in upper respiratory tract infection and found that participants who were unable to suppress their cough were significantly more excited, feeble, clumsy, incompetent, sad, antagonistic and had significantly greater scores for obsessional symptoms. This group indicated they required more effort to control their cough than the group who did not cough, and that this was not due to cold symptom severity. The authors suggested that these individuals might have a lower threshold at which voluntary behaviour, such as coughing, is deemed necessary.

Reflexive mechanisms underlying cough control are stronger than the voluntary mechanisms.[14] It could be assumed, therefore, that despite the potential for individuals to develop voluntary control over their cough, in many cases reflexive control of cough could predominate over cortical control. This theory provides a sound theoretical platform from which voluntary control of the cough in chronic refractory cough may be explored.

The relative involvement of cortical control in cough varies from having no influence on the cough response, such as when food or fluid enters the lungs, to having complete control of the cough response, for example when used as a means of communicating. Eccles[15] argued that cough in upper respiratory tract infection is a combination of both reflexive and voluntary components. Cortical involvement in chronic refractory cough may be demonstrated in patients who report deliberate coughing that is produced in response to a sensation of irritation and an urge to cough. Sensation of the urge to cough involves the cerebral cortex and deliberate cough appears to be related to this feeling.[16]

Reducing laryngeal irritation

The speech pathology intervention program described in Chapter 9, reduces stimulation of cough receptors and subsequently reduces the frequency of coughing. For example, decreased oral breathing improves filtration, humidification and warming of the air that might subsequently reduce laryngeal irritation in chronic refractory cough.[17] Hydration is a critical component of the vocal hygiene training. Several studies have found a beneficial effect on the larynx of adequate hydration,[18] including attenuating or delaying elevation of phonation threshold pressure,[19,20] and increasing resistance of the vocal folds to injury.[21,22] Improved hydration may reduce the effort required to initiate phonation, resulting in less stimulation of the cough receptors. Reduced cough episodes following treatment may decrease the rate and degree of stimulation of cough receptors, thus breaking the reciprocal cycle of the cough.

There is evidence that reflux episodes can occur as a result of cough paroxysms themselves.[23] It is possible that decreased coughing indirectly reduces lower esophageal sphincter opening associated with cough, thereby reducing reflux episodes that could potentially trigger further coughing.

Treatment can increase the patient's awareness of laryngeal irritation, which may provide more opportunity for them to employ cough suppression techniques. It is hypothesised that some individuals have mild irritation about which they are unaware and that, if prolonged or exacerbated, could trigger coughing. Speech pathology intervention teaches patients to anticipate a cough and then implement a strategy to suppress the cough.[11,24-26] In addition, identification and avoidance of triggers in the initial phases of intervention maximises the opportunity for cough control.

Treatment of coexisting Paradoxical Vocal Fold Movement

Speech pathology intervention targets underlying paradoxical vocal fold movement in some patients with chronic refractory cough. Breathing exercises for paradoxical vocal fold movement are designed to reduce laryngeal tension, promote a more rhythmic pattern of respiration and avoid tension associated with inspiration.[4] In these cases, the intervention could be presumed to be targeting the underlying cause of the cough.

Treatment of coexisting dysphonia

Although targeted voice therapy programs may be required for some patients with chronic refractory cough and paradoxical vocal fold movement, improvement in vocal quality can also occur following speech pathology treatment for chronic refractory cough.[27] Hypothesised mechanisms for improved vocal quality are summarized in Figure 13.1. It is possible that aberrant vocal quality is integral to the condition of chronic refractory cough and that effective treatment of cough will improve vocal function. Another possibility is that vocal fold oedema caused by repeated coughing resolves after effective treatment of chronic refractory cough. However, systematic studies of endoscopic evaluation of the larynx before and after treatment would be needed to confirm this hypothesis. A reduction in lower esophageal sphincter opening and subsequent reflux episodes, along with a reduction in cough episodes themselves, could reduce laryngeal irritation and vocal fold oedema, thus improving voice quality. Increased hydration could lower phonation threshold pressure and reduce the risk of laryngeal injury.[19] Voice quality might also improve due to reduced laryngeal irritation and cough reflex sensitivity. These factors can cause laryngeal tension in patients with chronic refractory cough as an attempted protective mechanism that subsequently manifests as impaired voice quality.[28,29] Cough

211

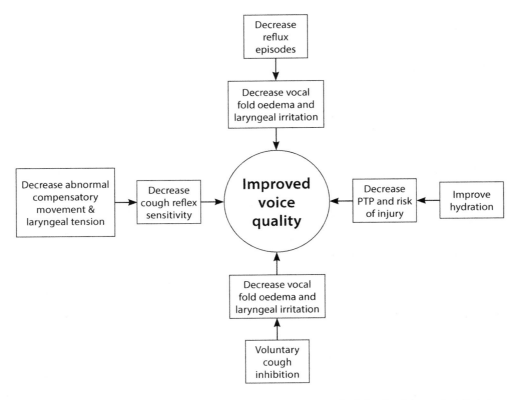

Figure 13.1: Possible mechanisms to explain improvement in voice quality following the speech pathology treatment. PTP = Phonation threshold pressure.

reflex sensitivity and laryngeal irritation reduce following treatment,[30,31] which could manifest as improved vocal fold closure and regularity of vocal fold vibration, thereby reducing features such as breathiness, roughness and strain.

Decreased coughing following intervention may lower anxiety in some patients, resulting in reduced extrinsic laryngeal muscle tension and associated vocal qualities, such as strain. Although anxiety is not necessarily a prevalent feature in many patients with chronic refractory cough, it may be relevant for some individuals. Physiological factors associated with voice quality, such as vocal fold closure and regularity of vocal fold vibration, could improve following intervention, whereas factors associated with pitch, such as subglottic pressure and length, mass and tension of the vocal folds, may remain unaffected.

It has been hypothesised that breathy voice quality and shorter closed phase of vocal fold vibration in patients with chronic refractory cough, could be due to attempts to reduce stimulation of the cough receptors during phonation that trigger coughing. Successful treatment of the cough could be associated with a

decreased tendency to avoid stimulation of the cough receptors during phonation, thereby reducing breathy and strained vocal qualities. However the lack of
significant change in the duration of closed phase following speech pathology
treatment,[27] does not support this hypothesis.

Reprogramming maladaptive responses

Speech pathology techniques for chronic refractory cough reprogram maladaptive central nervous system responses to the laryngeal irritation.[32] These exercises are designed to inhibit maladaptive responses, such as paradoxical vocal
fold movement, laryngospasm, constriction during phonation and cough and
help to redirect the patient's attention to alternative regions in the body, such
as the abdomen and face. In this process, motor learning principles are used to
change the undesirable muscle response patterns, such as coughing or increased
laryngeal muscle tension, to incoming stimuli. Altering response patterns by
reducing postural muscle tension and learning specific exercises will eventually
reduce symptoms of cough and laryngeal constriction.[32]

Placebo effect

Any active treatment will contain a placebo response.[33] This response has two
components (1) a nonspecific component which involves natural recovery, and
(2) a true placebo. The placebo effect in cough treatment is substantial in studies of antitussives,[15,34] and is particularly important to consider in behavioural
interventions. Eccles[35] proposed that the perceived placebo effect could be due
to a combination of the physiological effects of the placebo intervention, the
true placebo effect, and non-specific aspects such as spontaneous recovery over
time, or rest. The physiological effect of antitussive medication includes the
sugar content of cough mixture that encourages saliva production and swallowing, and stimulates sensory nerve endings in the epipharynx, thereby inhibiting the cough reflex. These physiological effects could be more important than
any pharmacological effect.[35] The true placebo effect depends upon the patient's
belief in the effectiveness of treatment and the attitude of the patient towards
the therapist, and might influence cough via a psychoneuropharmacological
response that releases endogenous active materials.[15]

Placebos may have a negative effect if the patient believes treatment is
harmful.[33] This concept is particularly relevant in speech pathology treatment of chronic refractory cough. Some patients referred for speech pathology

management believe it is harmful to suppress their cough. While they may be happy to practice the cough suppression exercises during asymptomatic periods, they may be reluctant to use these strategies to inhibit any cough episodes. This belief can have a negative effect on treatment and needs to be resolved before a successful outcome can be reached.

Summary

There is strong evidence for the efficacy of speech pathology intervention for patients with chronic refractory cough. The treatment results in improved quality of life, reduced cough frequency, reduced cough reflex sensitivity, and reduced urge to cough. The treatment also leads to improvements in auditory perceptual voice quality and acoustic voice measures. Mechanisms underlying these improvements include improved cough reflex sensitivity, improved voluntary control of cough, reduced laryngeal irritation, treatment of coexisting dysphonia and paradoxical vocal fold movement, and reprograming maladaptive responses. Speech pathology treatment is therefore important in the management of patients with chronic refractory cough.

References

1. Gay M, Blager F, Bartsch K, Emery C. Psychogenic habit cough: Review and case reports. *Journal of Child Psychiatry*. 1987;48(12):483–6.

2. Blager F, Gay M, Wood R. Voice therapy techniques adapted to treatment of habit cough: Pilot study. *Journal of Communication Disorders*. 1988;21:393–400.

3. Vertigan A. Speech pathology management of chronic cough. *Acquiring Knowledge in Speech Language and Hearing*. 2001;3(2):62–6.

4. Murry T, Tabaee A, Aviv J. Respiratory retraining of refractory cough and laryngopharyngeal reflux in patients with paradoxical vocal fold movement disorder. *The Laryngoscope*. 2004;114(8):1341–5.

5. Murry T, Branski R, Yu K, *et al*. Laryngeal sensory deficits in patients with chronic cough and paradoxical vocal fold movement disorder. *The Laryngoscope*. 2010;120:1576–81.

6. Vertigan A, Theodoros D, Gibson PG, Winkworth A. Efficacy of speech pathology management for chronic cough: a randomised placebo controlled trial of treatment efficacy. *Thorax*. 2006;61(12):1065–9.

7. Chung K. The clinical and pathophysiological challenge of cough. In: Chung K, Widdicome J, Boushey H (eds). *Cough: Causes, Mechanisms and Therapy*. Melbourne: Blackwell Publishing; 2003.

8. McGarvey L. Idiopathic chronic cough: A real disease or a failure of diagnosis? *Cough*. 2005;1: 9.

9. Young EC, Brammer C, Owen E, *et al*. The effect of mindfulness meditation on cough reflex sensitivity. *Thorax*. 2009;64(11):993–8.

10. Ryan N, Vertigan A, Gibson P. Chronic cough and laryngeal dysfunction improve with specific treatment of cough and paradoxical vocal fold movement. *Cough*. 2009;5:4.

11. Andrianopoulous M, Gallivan G, Gallivan K. PVCM, PVCD, EPL and Irritable Larynx Syndrome: What are we talking about and how do we treat it? *Journal of Voice*. 2000;14(4):607–18.

12. Lee P, Cotterill-Jones C, Eccles R. Voluntary control of cough. *Pulmonary Pharmacology & Therapeutics*. 2002;15(3):317–20.

13. Hutchings H, Eccles R, Smith A, Jawad M. Voluntary cough suppression as an indication of symptom severity in upper respiratory tract infections. *European Respiratory Journal*. 1993;6:1449–54.

14. Altman K, Simpson C, Amin M, *et al*. Cough and paradoxical vocal fold motion. *Otolaryngology Head & Neck Surgery*. 2002;127(6):501–11.

15. Eccles R. Placebo effects of antitussive treatments on cough associated with acute upper respiratory tract infection. In: Chung K, Widdicome J, Boushey H (eds). *Cough: Causes, Mechanisms and Therapy*. Melbourne: Blackwell Publishing; 2003.

16. Widdicombe J, Fontana G. Cough: what's in a name? *European Respiratory Journal*. 2006;28(1):10–15.

17. Guerra S, Sherrill DL, Baldacci S, *et al*. Rhinitis is an independent risk factor for developing cough apart from colds among adults. *Allergy*. 2005;60(3):343–9.

18. Casper J, Murry T. Voice therapy methods in dysphonia. *Otolaryngologic Clinics of North America*. 2000;33(5):983–1002.

19. Verdolini K, Titze I, Druker D. Changes in phonation threshold pressure with induced conditions of hydration. *Journal of Voice*. 1990;4:142–51.

20. Solomon NP, DiMattia MS. Effects of a vocally fatiguing task and systemic hydration on phonation threshold pressure. *Journal of Voice*. 2000;14(3):341–62.

21. Titze I. Heat generation in the vocal folds and its possible effectg on vocal endurance. In: Lawrence VE (ed). *Transcripts of the Tenth Symposium: Care of the Professional Voice*. New York, NY: The Voice Foundation; 1981. p. 52–9.

22. Verdolini-Marston K, Sandage M, Titze IR. Effect of hydration treatments on laryngeal nodules and polyps and related voice measures. *Journal of Voice*. 1994;8(1):30–47.

23. Ing AJ, Ngu MC, Breslin AB. Chronic persistent cough and gastro-oesophageal reflux. *Thorax*. 1991;46(7):479–83.

24. Martin R, Blager F, Gay M, Wood R. Paradoxical vocal fold motion in presumed asthmatics. *Seminars in Respiratory Medicine*. 1987;8(4):332–7.

25. Fulcher R, Cellucci T. Case formulation and behavioural treatment of chronic cough. *Journal of Behavior Therapy and Experimental Psychiatry*. 1997;28(4):291–6.

26. Mastrovich J, Greenberger P. Psychogenic cough in adults: A report of two cases and review of the literature. *Allergy and Asthma Proceedings*. 2002;23(1):27–33.

27. Vertigan A, Theodoros D, Winkworth A, Gibson P. A comparison of two approaches to the treatment of chronic cough: Perceptual acoustic and electroglottographic outcomes. *Journal of Voice*. 2008;22(5):581–9.

28. Choudry NB, Fuller RW. Sensitivity of the cough reflex in patients with chronic cough. *European Respiratory Journal*. 1992;5(3):296–300.

29. Ryan N, Gibson P. Cough reflex hypersensitivity and upper airway hyperresponsiveness in vocal cord dysfunction with chronic cough. *Respirology*. 2006;11 (Suppl 2):A48.

30. Ryan NM, Vertigan AE, Bone S, Gibson PG. Cough reflex sensitivity improves with speech language pathology management of refractory chronic cough. *Cough*. 2010;6(1):1–8.

31. Vertigan AE, Bone SL, Gibson PG. Development and validation of the Newcastle laryngeal hypersensitivity questionnaire. *Cough*. 2014;10(1):1.

32. Stemple J, Fry L. *Voice Therapy: Clinical Case Studies*. 3rd edn. San Diego, CA: Plural Publishing; 2009.

33. Eccles R. The power of the placebo. *Current Allergy and Asthma Reports*. 2007;7(2):100–4.

34. Smith J, Owen E, Earis J, Woodcock A. Effect of codeine on objective measurement of cough in chronic obstructive pulmonary disease. *Journal of Allergy and Clinical Immunology*. 2006;117(4):831–5.

35. Eccles R. Mechanisms of the placebo effect of sweet cough syrups. *Respiratory, Physiology and Neurobiology*. 2005;152(3):340–8.

Appendix 1: Chronic cough and PVFM case history form

Patient name: _____ MRN: _____ DOB: _____

Date assessed: _____ Referred by: _____ Reason: _____

Main referring diagnosis: _____

Presenting problem (as reported by patient)	
Symptoms	Cough: *Yes / No* Breathing: *Yes / No* *(e.g. difficulty inspiring air, shortness of breath on exercise)* Voice: *Yes / No* Upper airway: *Yes / No* *(e.g. swallowing problems, globus)*
Onset / Duration / Progression	
Cough symptoms	**Triggers:** Smoke: *Yes / No / NA* Stress/anxiety: *Yes / No / NA* Fumes/bleach/aerosols: *Yes / No / NA* Sensation in throat: *Yes / No / NA* Exercise: *Yes / No / NA* Eating: *Yes / No / NA* Talking/laughing/telephone: *Yes / No / NA* Perfume: *Yes / No / NA* Cold air/air conditioning: *Yes / No / NA* Humidity: *Yes / No / NA* Shortness of Breath: *Yes / No / NA* Other: _____ **Urge to cough:** Urge to cough magnitude rating: _____ Sensation before coughing: _____ Cough description: *Dry / Moist / Other* Where initiated: *Throat / Chest / Both / Unsure* Cough deliberately: *Never / Occasionally / Frequently* Pattern of cough: *Continuous / Bouts / Other* Strategies used to control cough: _____ Patient concern over cough: _____ Sensation after cough: _____

PVFM symptoms	Inspiration > Expiration:	Yes / No
	Throat tightness:	Yes / No
	Upper chest tightness:	Yes / No
	Stridor:	Yes / No
	Triggers: _____	
	Choking, suffocation, strangulation:	Yes / No
	Effectiveness of inhaled bronchodilators:	Effective / Ineffective
	Rapid onset of symptoms :	Yes / No
	Rapid resolution of symptoms:	Yes / No
	Numbness:	Yes / No
	Dizziness:	Yes / No
	Patient concern over breathing: _____	
Voice symptoms		
Swallowing symptoms		

Medical history	REFLUX:	Yes / No
	Previous reflux treatment? _____	
	Last time reviewed? _____	
	Treatment effective for reflux:	Yes / No/ Partial
	Treatment effective for cough:	Yes / No / Partial
	ASTHMA:	Yes / No
	If yes, how diagnosed? _____	
	Previous asthma treatment?	Yes / No Last time reviewed? _____
	Treatment effective for asthma?	Yes / No / Partial
	Treatment effective for cough?	Yes / No / Partial
	RHINITIS:	Yes / No
	Previous rhinitis treatment?	Yes / No Type: _____
	Treatment effective for rhinitis?	Yes / No / Partial
	Treatment effective for cough?	Yes / No / Partial
	Smoking?	Yes / No / Ceased

218

	ACE inhibitor: *Yes / No / Ceased* If ceased, any impact on cough? *Yes / No*
	ENT review: *Yes / No* Result: _____
	Saline challenge test: *Yes / No* Result: _____
	Chest radiograph?: *Yes / No* Result: _____
	Obstructive sleep apnoea? *Yes / No* Snoring? *Yes /No*
	Other medical history
	Medications
Mental health and emotional issues	

Social history	

Vocal use and vocally traumatic behaviours	Shouting:	*Yes / No*	Loud talking:	*Yes / No*
	Screaming:	*Yes / No*	Vocal noises:	*Yes / No*
	Coughing:	*Yes / No*	Throat clearing:	*Yes / No*
	Vocal use:	*Limited / Moderate / Extensive*		
	Professional voice user:	*Yes / No*		
	Singer:	*Yes / No*		

Vocal hygeine	Water intake: _____
	Smoking: *Yes / No*
	Alcohol: _____
	Drugs: _____
	Caffeine: _____
	Breathing Route: *Mouth / Nose / Both / Unsure*
	Poor sleep : *Yes / No*
	Exposure to fumes: *Yes / No*

Appendix 2: Symptom frequency and severity rating

Name: _____ Date: _____

Please rate how <u>FREQUENTLY</u> the following symptoms have occurred in the last week

1. **Difficulty breathing**   *(circle one)*

    All of the time 5

    Most of the time 4

    A good bit of the time 3

    A little of the time 2

    None of the time 1

2. **Cough**   *(circle one)*

    All of the time 5

    Most of the time 4

    A good bit of the time 3

    A little of the time 2

    None of the time 1

3. **Throat clearing**   *(circle one)*

    All of the time 5

    Most of the time 4

    A good bit of the time 3

    A little of the time 2

    None of the time 1

4. **Voice difficulty** *(circle one)*

    All of the time 5

    Most of the time 4

    A good bit of the time 3

    A little of the time 2

    None of the time 1

5. **Shortness of breath** *(circle one)*

    All of the time 5

    Most of the time 4

    A good bit of the time 3

    A little of the time 2

    None of the time 1

6. **Throat tightness** *(circle one)*

    All of the time 5

    Most of the time 4

    A good bit of the time 3

    A little of the time 2

    None of the time 1

7. **A sensation of something in the throat** *(circle one)*

    All of the time 5

    Most of the time 4

    A good bit of the time 3

    A little of the time 2

    None of the time 1

8. **Difficulty swallowing** *(circle one)*

    All of the time 5

    Most of the time 4

    A good bit of the time 3

    A little of the time 2

    None of the time 1

9. **Dry mouth or throat** *(circle one)*

    All of the time 5

    Most of the time 4

    A good bit of the time 3

    A little of the time 2

    None of the time 1

10. **Voice sounds deeper** *(circle one)*

    All of the time 5

    Most of the time 4

    A good bit of the time 3

    A little of the time 2

    None of the time 1

11. **I lose my voice** *(circle one)*

    All of the time 5

    Most of the time 4

    A good bit of the time 3

    A little of the time 2

    None of the time 1

12. **I feel like I'm going to choke or gag when I eat or drink** *(circle one)*

    All of the time 5

    Most of the time 4

    A good bit of the time 3

    A little of the time 2

    None of the time 1

13. **Feelings of anxiety** *(circle one)*

    All of the time 5

    Most of the time 4

    A good bit of the time 3

    A little of the time 2

    None of the time 1

14. Voice feels tired   *(circle one)*

All of the time 5

Most of the time 4

A good bit of the time 3

A little of the time 2

None of the time 1

15. I can't speak as loudly   *(circle one)*

All of the time 5

Most of the time 4

A good bit of the time 3

A little of the time 2

None of the time 1

16 . Difficulty breathing in   *(circle one)*

All of the time 5

Most of the time 4

A good bit of the time 3

A little of the time 2

None of the time 1

17. Difficulty breathing out   *(circle one)*

All of the time 5

Most of the time 4

A good bit of the time 3

A little of the time 2

None of the time 1

Please rate how <u>SEVERE</u> the following symptoms have been in the last week

1. Breathing difficulty   *(circle one)*

Most severe discomfort ever 5

Moderate discomfort 4

Mild discomfort 3

Barely perceptible 2

Absent, none at all 1

2. Coughing *(circle one)*

Most severe discomfort ever	5
Moderate discomfort	4
Mild discomfort	3
Barely perceptible	2
Absent, none at all	1

3. Throat clearing *(circle one)*

Most severe discomfort ever	5
Moderate discomfort	4
Mild discomfort	3
Barely perceptible	2
Absent, none at all	1

4. Voice problems *(circle one)*

Most severe discomfort ever	5
Moderate discomfort	4
Mild discomfort	3
Barely perceptible	2
Absent, none at all	1

5. Other throat symptoms *(circle one)*

Most severe discomfort ever	5
Moderate discomfort	4
Mild discomfort	3
Barely perceptible	2
Absent, none at all	1

How did these symptoms affect your day to day activity? *Please circle*

Not limited – have done all the activities that I want to	1
Mildly limited – few activities not done	2
Moderately limited – several activities not done	3
Very limited	4
Severely limited – most activities not done	5

Of all these symptoms, which is the most annoying?

224

Appendix 3: Leicester Cough Questionnaire

(Birring et al., 2003)

1. **In the last 2 weeks, have you had chest or stomach pains as a result of your cough?** *(circle one)*

   All of the time 1

   Most of the time 2

   A good bit of the time 3

   Some of the time 4

   A little of the time 5

   Hardly any of the time 6

   None of the time 7

2. **In the last 2 weeks, have you been bothered by sputum (phlegm) production when you cough?** *(circle one)*

   Every time 1

   Most times 2

   Several times 3

   Sometimes 4

   Occasionally 5

   Rarely 6

   Never 7

3. **In the last 2 weeks, have you been tired because of your cough?** *(circle one)*

All of the time	1
Most of the time	2
A good bit of the time	3
Some of the time	4
A little of the time	5
Hardly any of the time	6
None of the time	7

4. **In the last 2 weeks, have you felt in control of your cough?** *(circle one)*

None of the time	1
Hardly any of the time	2
A little of the time	3
Some of the time	4
A good bit of the time	5
Most of the time	6
All of the time	7

5. **How often during the last 2 weeks have you felt embarrassed by your coughing?**

(circle one)

All of the time	1
Most of the time	2
A good bit of the time	3
Some of the time	4
A little of the time	5
Hardly any of the time	6
None of the time	7

6. **In the last 2 weeks, my cough has made me feel anxious** *(circle one)*

All of the time	1
Most of the time	2
A good bit of the time	3
Some of the time	4
A little of the time	5
Hardly any of the time	6
None of the time	7

7. **In the last 2 weeks, my cough has interfered with my job, or other daily tasks**

(circle one)

All of the time	1
Most of the time	2
A good bit of the time	3
Some of the time	4
A little of the time	5
Hardly any of the time	6
None of the time	7

8. **In the last 2 weeks, I felt that my cough interfered with the overall enjoyment of my life**

(circle one)

All of the time	1
Most of the time	2
A good bit of the time	3
Some of the time	4
A little of the time	5
Hardly any of the time	6
None of the time	7

9. **In the last 2 weeks, exposure to paints or fumes has made me cough**

(circle one)

All of the time	1
Most of the time	2
A good bit of the time	3
Some of the time	4
A little of the time	5
Hardly any of the time	6
None of the time	7

10. **In the last 2 weeks, has your cough disturbed your sleep?** *(circle one)*

All of the time 1

Most of the time 2

A good bit of the time 3

Some of the time 4

A little of the time 5

Hardly any of the time 6

None of the time 7

11. **In the last 2 weeks, how many times a day have you had coughing bouts?**

(circle one)

All of the time (continuously) 1

Most times during the day 2

Several times during the day 3

Some times during the day 4

Occasionally through the day 5

Rarely 6

None 7

12. **In the last 2 weeks, my cough has made me feel frustrated** *(circle one)*

All of the time 1

Most of the time 2

A good bit of the time 3

Some of the time 4

A little of the time 5

Hardly any of the time 6

None of the time 7

13. **In the last 2 weeks, my cough has made me feel fed up** .... *(circle one)*

All of the time 1

Most of the time 2

A good bit of the time 3

Some of the time 4

A little of the time 5

Hardly any of the time 6

None of the time 7

14. **In the last 2 weeks, have you suffered from a hoarse voice as a result of your cough?** *(circle one)*

All of the time 1
Most of the time 2
A good bit of the time 3
Some of the time 4
A little of the time 5
Hardly any of the time 6
None of the time 7

15. **In the last 2 weeks, have you had a lot of energy?** *(circle one)*

None of the time 1
Hardly any of the time 2
A little of the time 3
Some of the time 4
A good bit of the time 5
Most of the time 6
All of the time 7

16. **In the last 2 weeks, have you worried that your cough may indicate serious illness?** *(circle one)*

All of the time 1
Most of the time 2
A good bit of the time 3
Some of the time 4
A little of the time 5
Hardly any of the time 6
None of the time 7

229

17. **In the last 2 weeks, have you been concerned that other people think something is wrong with you, because of your cough?** *(circle one)*

All of the time 1
Most of the time 2
A good bit of the time 3
Some of the time 4
A little of the time 5
Hardly any of the time 6
None of the time 7

18. **In the last 2 weeks, my cough has interrupted conversation or telephone calls**
(circle one)

Every time 1
Most of the time 2
A good bit of the time 3
Some of the time 4
A little of the time 5
Hardly any of the time 6
None of the time 7

19. **In the last 2 weeks, I feel that my cough has annoyed my partner, family or friends** *(circle one)*

Every time I cough 1
Most times when I cough 2
Several times when I cough 3
Sometimes when I cough 4
Occasionally when I cough 5
Rarely 6
Never 7

Thank you for completing this questionnaire.

Appendix 4: Newcastle Laryngeal Hypersensitivity Questionnaire

Please circle the answer that best describes you currently. Be sure to select only one response:

Example: I watch television:

All of the time	Most of the time	A good bit of the time	Some of the time	A little of the time	Hardly any of the time	None of the time
1	2	3	(4)	5	6	7

---

1. There is an abnormal sensation in my throat: (O)

All of the time	Most of the time	A good bit of the time	Some of the time	A little of the time	Hardly any of the time	None of the time
1	2	3	4	5	6	7

---

2. I feel phlegm and mucous in my throat: (TT)

All of the time	Most of the time	A good bit of the time	Some of the time	A little of the time	Hardly any of the time	None of the time
1	2	3	4	5	6	7

---

3. I have a pain in my throat: (P/Th)

All of the time	Most of the time	A good bit of the time	Some of the time	A little of the time	Hardly any of the time	None of the time
1	2	3	4	5	6	7

---

4. I have a sensation of something stuck in my throat: (O)

All of the time	Most of the time	A good bit of the time	Some of the time	A little of the time	Hardly any of the time	None of the time
1	2	3	4	5	6	7

5. My throat is blocked: (O)

All of the time	Most of the time	A good bit of the time	Some of the time	A little of the time	Hardly any of the time	None of the time
1	2	3	4	5	6	7

6. My throat feels tight: (O)

All of the time	Most of the time	A good bit of the time	Some of the time	A little of the time	Hardly any of the time	None of the time
1	2	3	4	5	6	7

7. There is an irritation in my throat: (O)

All of the time	Most of the time	A good bit of the time	Some of the time	A little of the time	Hardly any of the time	None of the time
1	2	3	4	5	6	7

8. I have a sensation of something pushing on my chest: (P/Th)

All of the time	Most of the time	A good bit of the time	Some of the time	A little of the time	Hardly any of the time	None of the time
1	2	3	4	5	6	7

9. I have a sensation of something pressing on my throat: (O)

All of the time	Most of the time	A good bit of the time	Some of the time	A little of the time	Hardly any of the time	None of the time
1	2	3	4	5	6	7

10. There is a feeling of constriction as though needing to inhale a large amount of air (O)

All of the time	Most of the time	A good bit of the time	Some of the time	A little of the time	Hardly any of the time	None of the time
1	2	3	4	5	6	7

11. Food catches when I eat or drink: (O)

All of the time	Most of the time	A good bit of the time	Some of the time	A little of the time	Hardly any of the time	None of the time
1	2	3	4	5	6	7

12. There is a tickle in my throat: (TT)

All of the time	Most of the time	A good bit of the time	Some of the time	A little of the time	Hardly any of the time	None of the time
1	2	3	4	5	6	7

13. There is an itch in my throat: (TT)

All of the time	Most of the time	A good bit of the time	Some of the time	A little of the time	Hardly any of the time	None of the time
1	2	3	4	5	6	7

14. I have a hot or burning sensation in my throat: (P/Th)

All of the time	Most of the time	A good bit of the time	Some of the time	A little of the time	Hardly any of the time	None of the time
1	2	3	4	5	6	7

Office use only:

TOTAL OBSTRUCTION (O) SCORE ☐   AVERAGE OBSTRUCTION SCORE = (TOTAL SCORE/8) ☐

TOTAL PAIN/THERMAL (P/Th) SCORE ☐   AVERAGE PAIN/THERMAL SCORE = (TOTAL SCORE/3) ☐

TOTAL THROAT TICKLE (TT) SCORE ☐   AVERAGE THROAT TICKLE SCORE = (TOTAL SCORE/3) ☐

TOTAL LHQ SCORE = (AVERAGE OBSTRUCTION + AVERAGE PAIN/THERMAL + AVERAGE THROAT TICKLE) ☐

Appendix 5: Chronic chough/ paradoxical vocal fold movement assessment

Circle appropriate information and add comment.

Patient name: DOB: Date: SP: MRN:

Oromusculature	Cranial nerve involvement: Oral cavity:		
Swallowing	**Swallowing:**	*Normal / Abnormal*	
	Timed Swallow Test: ___ seconds for ___ ml = ___ ml/second [normal range > 10 ml/second]		
Respiration	**Habitual breathing:** Route:	*Oral / Nasal / Both*	
	Breathing pattern:	*Clavicular / Thoracic / Diaphragmatic / Abdominal*	
	Breathing difficulty: Cycle:	*Inspiration / Expiration / Both*	
	Timing:	*At rest / Physical activity / Other*	
	Struggling for air:	*Yes / No*	
	Effortful inhalation:	*Yes / No*	
	Stridor:	*Yes / No*	
	Breath holding:	*Yes / No* (If 'yes' note activity)	
	Respiratory rate:	_____	
Cough (Observe)	**Cough during session:**	*Dry / Moist / Not observed / Other*	
	Throat clearing during session:	*Present / Absent*	
	Pattern of cough:	*Intermittent / Continuous*	
	Cough triggered by voice assessment tasks: *Yes / No*		
	Attempts to suppress cough and effectiveness of attempts: _____		
Posture / Tension	**Neck and shoulder tension:**		
	During quiet respiration	*Present / Absent*	
	During phonation	*Present / Absent*	
	Excess extrinsic laryngeal muscle tension:		
	Location:	*Thyrohyoid / Suprahyoid / Mandible / Absent*	
	When present:	*At rest / Inspiration / Expiration / Initiation of phonation*	
	General body tension:	*Torso / Limbs / Absent*	
	Posture: _____		

Voice / Speech	**Reading aloud, monologue, or conversation**
	Coordination of respiration and phonation: _____
	Auditory perceptual voice analysis of pitch, loudness, and quality:
	CAPE-V Rating Overall Severity: ____ / 100
	Articulation, language, resonance, fluency: _____
	Non-instrumental voice assessment tasks
	Pitch range [Scale or glide task]: _____
	Loudness range [Phonate and minimum and maximum volumes]: _____
	Fatigue [Count from 1 to 50. Observe coordination of respiration and phonation and fatigue, e.g. does the voice deteriorate with increased talking] _____
	Prolongation time /s/: _____
	Maximum phonation time: _____
	Laryngeal diadachokinesis: _____
	Tests of vocal fold swelling: [soft sustained /i/; repetition /hi/; soft ascending glide; soft high singing of "happy birthday"] _____
	Articulation/language/fluency: _____
	Phonotraumatic behaviours [e.g. throat clearing; hard glottal attacks; laryngeal focus of resonance; reduced breath support; inappropriate pitch or loudness]: _____
	Voice Stress Test: _____
Motivation	
Instrumental testing	Completed / not completed

Appendix 6: Urge to cough test

John Hunter Hospital, Speech Pathology Department

Patient: MRN: DOB:

Diabetes   *Yes / No*

		UTC rating	Cough count	Comments
Baseline	Baseline			
Respiration	Deep inspiration			
Exercise	Exercise (5 min)			
Phonation	Reading (1 min) Maximum Phonation Time (3 trials) Scale task Loudness Fatigue (1–50) Voice Stress Test (2 min)			
Inhaled	Perfume Soap powder			
Swallowing	Biscuit Timed Swallow Test			
Relieving Strategies	Sip water Quiet breathing (1 min) Suck on lolly (1 min) Chewing gum (1 min) Honey End of session			

Appendix 7: Capsaicin cough reflex sensitivity test

John Hunter Hospital and Hunter Medical Research Institute

Patient:　　　　　　　MRN:　　　　　　　DOB:

Baseline spirometry	Predicted	Observed	% Predicted or %FEV1/FVC
FEV_1			
FVC			
FEV_1 / FVC			
FIF_{50}			
Inspiratory time			
Urge-to-cough			

Capsaicin challenge	No. of coughs	Urge-to-cough	Summary
0.98 uMol			
Saline			
1.96 uMol			CT =
3.92 uMol			
7.84 uMol			C5 =
15.7 uMol			
31.4 uMol			
62.7 uMol			
125.4 uMol			UTC at baseline
250.9 uMol			UTC at C5 =
500.0 uMol			

End of challenge spirometry	Observed	% Predicted or %FEV1/FVC
FEV_1		
FVC		
FEV_1 / FVC		
FIF_{50}		
Inspiratory time		
Post challenge urge-to-cough		

Appendix 8: Speech pathology treatment for chronic cough: education material

Patient: _____

Speech Pathologist: _____ Date: _____

This handout is specifically designed for patients who experience chronic cough and excessive throat clearing. It can be helpful to understand the nature of cough when you are attempting to control the cough.

The following diagram (Figure 1) shows a picture of the larynx which is sometimes referred to as the 'voice box'. The vocal folds (Figure 2), which are part of the larynx, open when you breathe so that air can pass freely in and out of the lungs. The vocal folds close when you speak. Air passes through the vocal folds causing them to vibrate and produce voice. When you cough, or clear your throat, the vocal folds slam together. Frequent coughing and throat clearing can be very damaging to the vocal folds. When you swallow, your vocal folds also close but they do so with a gentle movement. They close to prevent food, liquid or saliva entering your airway.

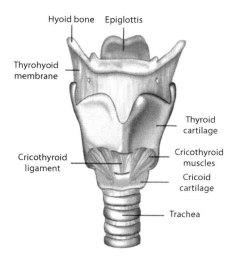

Figure 1: The larynx.

239

Six facts about cough

Fact one. A cough can be triggered by irritation of larynx, throat, or breathing tubes leading to the lungs. A large number of people also cough deliberately in response to irritation in the throat. Coughing can become a viscous cycle where irritation leads to coughing, coughing causes more irritation, and irritation leads to more coughing.

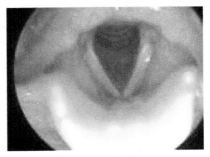

Figure 2: The vocal folds in open position.

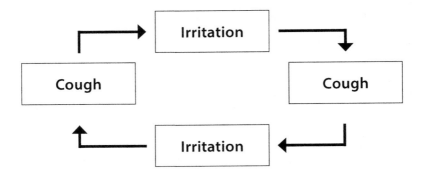

Fact two. A cough protects the body by clearing the lungs and tubes of things that irritate the body and secretions such as phlegm and mucous. Therefore, in some cases a cough can be beneficial. This is particularly true when you have swallowed food down the wrong way or when you have a chest infection.

Fact three. Your cough is not always necessary. In the case of chronic cough, the cough is often occurring in response to irritation rather than because anything needs to be cleared from your lungs or chest. In other words, there is no benefit to coughing. In fact, there are a lot of negative side-effects to coughing, such as increasing throat irritation and urinary incontinence.

> **The feeling is real but the need to cough is not.**
> **Dr. Florence Blager, 2003**

Fact four. Coughing is both automatic and under conscious control. Coughing, like everything else we do, is controlled by the brain. The brain is made up of many different sections (Figure 3). The bottom section, shown circled in grey, controls all the automatic functions of our body such as breathing and maintaining body temperature. This part of the brain is called the medulla and has an important role in cough. The top section of our brain, which is circled in white is responsible for conscious actions, for example walking, talking, driving a car, playing golf, thinking, etc. This section is called the cerebral cortex. Research has shown that the cerebral cortex is also activated during cough. So although coughing often occurs automatically, there is still an element of conscious con-

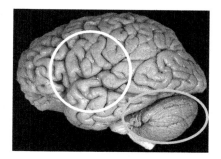

Figure 3: Control of cough.

trol. That is why we can suppress a cough at times and why we can cough deliberately. In speech pathology treatment we aim to strengthen your voluntary control of cough.

Fact five. The most common causes of cough are asthma, gastroesophageal reflux, post nasal drip, eosinophilic bronchitis, smoking, lung pathology and vocal cord dysfunction. In approximately 10% of patients, no cause can be found. Speech pathology intervention is designed for patients who (1) have no known cause for their cough, (2) have vocal cord dysfunction, and (3) have cough persisting despite treatment for asthma, rhinitis and gastroesophageal reflux.

Fact six. Medical treatment is effective for most people with chronic cough (Figure 4). In fact, 80% of patients with chronic cough are helped by medical treatment. However, 20% of people with chronic cough do not respond to medical treatment. In other words, for every 100 people with chronic cough, 80 will improve and 20 will not improve after medical treatment. Speech pathology treatment is designed for these individuals.

Two ways that speech pathology treatment can help your cough

1. **Increase conscious control over the cough.** Speech pathology treatment increases your ability to voluntarily control your cough. Although irritation may build up in the throat, it will eventually be possible for you to learn to control your cough. It is also possible to control or suppress the cough when you feel that something needs to be coughed up.

2. **Reduce the irritation that triggers coughing.** Speech pathology treatment also reduces the degree of irritation in your throat and airway. A cough is triggered once irritation builds up to a certain level. Increasing irritation can trigger a cough, whereas reducing irritation reduces coughing. So if the rate of irritation can be slowed, then a cough is less likely to be triggered.

Speech pathology treatment has been proven to be beneficial for people with chronic cough. A large study examined 87 patients with chronic cough that persisted despite extensive medical treatment. These patients were randomly selected to receive either the speech pathology treatment or a placebo intervention. Of those who received the speech pathology treatment, 88% improved, whereas 14% of those who received the placebo intervention improved (see Figure 5).

Medical treatment for cough

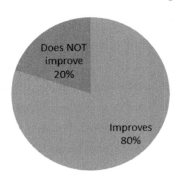

Outcomes of treatment

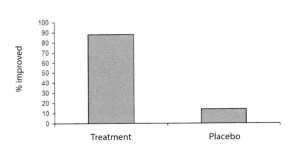

Figure 4: Outcomes of medical treatment for cough.

Figure 5: Outcomes of speech pathology treatment for chronic cough.

Appendix 9: Cough suppression swallow

John Hunter Hospital, Speech Pathology Department

The cough and swallow have similar mechanisms and therefore the swallow can replace a cough. You will need to become aware when a cough is about to occur. Replace the cough with a swallow even if you feel there is something you need to cough up. Swallow when you feel a sensation of a tickle in the throat. At the very first sign of a cough do an effortful swallow:

- with your hands pushed together, and
- with your head down towards your chest.

The cough suppression swallow can be performed:

- as dry swallow,
- with water, or
- with a non-medicated lolly.

Do the cough suppression swallow at the very FIRST sign of cough.

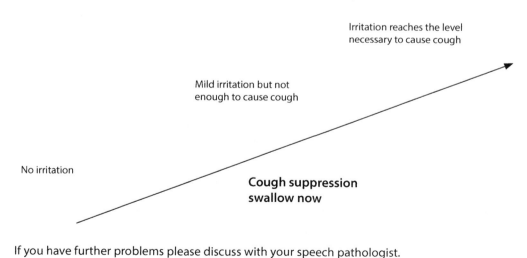

If you have further problems please discuss with your speech pathologist.

Speech Pathologist: _____

Telephone Number _____

Appendix 10: Seven ways to reduce irritation that causes coughing

Vocal hygiene strategies for chronic cough

Patient: _____

Speech Pathologist: _____   Date: _____

Reducing irritation in your throat and airway is an important component of treatment for chronic cough. Coughing is triggered once irritation builds up to a certain level. Increasing irritation can trigger a cough whereas reducing irritation reduces coughing. A cough is less likely to be triggered if the rate of irritation can be slowed. There are several strategies for reducing irritation, which are described below.

1.   Drink adequate quantities of water

If you are not well hydrated your vocal folds will have to work a lot harder whenever you talk. Drinking adequate water will also promote healing and reduce risk of injury. Many people with chronic cough are poorly hydrated.

- Aim to drink at least 2 litres of water a day and more during hot weather or exercise.
- Drink water frequently throughout the day, e.g. take small sips every 15 minutes.
- Drink water when your throat feels irritated rather than coughing and clearing your throat.
- If you do not like water try adding small amounts of lemon, lime or orange juice, mint leaves, and experiment with different temperatures.

2.   Avoid exposure to smoke

Smoking is irritating, damaging, and drying to the larynx. Smoking is one of the leading causes of cancer in the lungs and larynx. Reducing exposure to smoking and smoky environments can reduce irritation.

3. Breathe through your nose

Your nose has three important functions. Your nose

- warms the air,
- cleans the air, and
- humidifies the air.

Therefore, if you breathe through your nose the air will be warm, clean and moist when it reaches your throat and lungs. However if you breathe through your mouth, the air will be cold, dirty and dry. It is no surprise that cold, dry and dirty air causes irritation. Breathing through your nose will reduce irritation. It can be difficult to breathe through your nose if you are in the habit of mouth breathing. The best strategy is to breathe through your nose whenever you remember.

4. Minimise intake of dehydrating substances

Substances containing alcohol (e.g. wine, beer and spirits) and caffeine (e.g. tea, coffee, cola) are very drying and can increase irritation that leads to coughing. It would be ideal to eliminate or minimise these until you get your cough under control.

5. Lifestyle strategies for reflux

Reflux can be associated with cough. The following strategies are important if you have suspected reflux.

- Raise the head of your bed when sleeping. This reduces the chance of stomach acid reaching the level of the vocal folds while you are lying down. **Propping yourself up on cushions is not sufficient**.
- Reduce intake of foods that can trigger reflux such as chocolate, spicy food, fatty food, caffeine, and alcohol.
- Lose weight if you are overweight.
- Eat smaller meals rather than larger meals.
- Avoid eating or drinking before going to bed.

6. Inhale steam

Research has shown that inhaling steam adds moisture to the surface of your vocal folds. This promotes healing and reduces the risk of injury.

- Fill your kitchen sink with hot or boiling water.
- Breathe in the moist air or steam.

- Do not add anything to the water. Most substances that you add to the water will cause dryness and irritation.

7. Suck on non-medicated lozenges, chewing gum, or honey

Sucking on non-medicated lozenges causes you to produce more saliva and swallow more frequently, which can be very soothing to the throat. Avoid medicated cough lollipops; in particular, those which contain menthol can be drying to the throat and should be avoided. Similarly, chewing gum or swallowing whole teaspoons of honey increase the rate of swallowing and have a soothing effect.

Appendix 11: Treatment plan

Name: _____ Date: _____

Speech pathologist: _____

Assessment item	Possible treatment strategy (delete those that do not apply)
1. Reflux symtoms or increased RSI score	• Employ strategies to reduce reflux. • Raise head of bed. • Small frequent meals. • Reduce tight clothing. • Avoid eating before bed. • Diet modification. • Chewing gum.
2. Abnormalities identified during voice screening	• Consider need for voice therapy techniques.
3. Phonotraumatic behaviours	• Consider need for voice therapy.
4. Increased VHI score or voice symptom score	• Consider need for formal voice assessment.
5. Cough triggered by voice assessment	• More extensive voice assessment. • Direct voice therapy techniques. • Observe for features such as hard glottal attacks and laryngeal focus of resonance.
6. Urge to cough	• If present: Employ cough suppression technique (specify) at first urge to cough. • If absent: Rate urge to cough every 15 minutes and implement cough suppression strategy each time it rises over 2–3.

	• If absent: use cough suppression technique to interrupt rather than prevent cough.

7. Deliberate coughing	• Reduce deliberate coughing.
	• Respond to to cough urge by sipping water and swallowing phlegm.
	• Strategies to relieve uncomfortable throat sensation:
	  • Increase water intake and drink water to substitute cough.
	  • Suck non medicated lollies.
	  • Avoid laryngeal irritants.
	  • Avoid frequent throat clearing.
	  • Soothing products, e.g. non medicated lollies or teaspoons of honey.

8. Nocturnal cough	• Consider reflux strategies. • Water beside bed. • Encourage nasal breathing.
9. Pattern of coughing	If intermittent: • Increase awareness of throat irritation and implement strategies to suppress the cough at the first sign of irritation. If continuous: • Aim for a set symptom free period during the day and gradually extend duration.
10. Cough during session	• Set aside designated time to focus on suppressing cough • Attempt to suppress cough during the session.
11. Attempts to suppress cough & effectiveness of these attempts	• Reinforce attempts if present.
12. Throat clear during session	• Behaviour modification program for chronic refractory cough. For example, sipping water and increasing awareness.

13. Triggers	• Avoid or limit exposure.
	• Keep diary of specific triggers.
	• Specific triggers:
	  o Talking: may need voice therapy.
	  o Eating/drinking without oropharyngeal dysphagia: may be due to increased laryngeal sensitivity.
	  o Stress/anxiety: may require relaxation exercises. Con sider referral to mental health professional.
	  o Shortness of breath: ensure associated conditions such as asthma and paradoxical vocal fold movement are adequately managed.

14. PVFM symptoms	• Employ paradoxical vocal fold movement suppression techniques (specify) at first sign of breathing difficulty or tightness.
15. Severe paradoxical vocal fold movment episodes or cough syncope	• Emergency strategies for paradoxical vocal fold movement.
16. Habitual breathing pattern	• May need to work on relaxed breathing. • Tactile cues to reduce shoulder and neck tension. • Encourage nasal breathing.
17. Breathing difficulty	• Ensure optimal medical management including compliance with any asthma medications. • Refer for re-assessment if there is an exacerbation. • Assess for paradoxical vocal fold movement.
18. Stridor	• Assess for paradoxical vocal fold movement. • Is the patient able to change their breathing pattern with instruction?
19. Breath holding	• Draw attention to breath holding at rest and then during other activities. • Diary regarding breath holding events, e.g. when gardening, hanging out washing.

20. Poor hydration	• Increase water intake to two litres a day. • Sip water every 15 minutes. • Inhale steam. • Flavour water.
21. Exposed to laryngeal irritants	• Avoid or reduce alcohol. • Avoid smoking. • Avoid or reduce caffeine. • Promote nose breathing. • Reduce extensive talking. • Avoid cough lozenges. • Chewing gum / honey / non-medicated lozenges. • Consider referral to mental health professional. • Investigate and manage oropharyngeal dysphagia.
22. Possible anxiety or depression	• Consider referral to mental health professional.
23. Abnormalities in cranial nerve, dysphagia, or oro musculature assessment	• Investigate and manage oropharyngeal dysphagia.
24. Neck/shoulder tension	• Raise awareness of tension. • Inviting patient to 'notice' any tension while breathing. May need repeated advice. • Head neck stretches.
25. Extrinsic laryngeal muscle tension	• May need direct therapy to address this, e.g. neck/shoulder stretches, release of constriction similar to that provided in many voice therapy programs.
26. Patient motivation	• Reinforce current motivation. • Discuss motivation and implement strategies.

Plan:

1. **Therapy schedule:** (e.g. frequency)

2. **Symptom suppression exercises:**

3. **Implementation of symptom suppression exercises:** (e.g. at first sign of cough, in symptom free periods)

4. **Therapy goals:** For example:

   Identify precipitating sensation and substitute with strategy

   Reduce laryngeal irritation

   Improve symptom control

   Improve voice quality

   Improve efficiency of phonation

5. **Recommendations:**

Appendix 12: Laryngeal sensation diary

Implement your cough suppression strategy each time the urge to cough rating reaches 2 or above. Indicate the number which best describes your cough.

0	Nothing at all
0.5	Very, very weak (just noticeable)
1	Very weak
2	Weak
3	Moderate
4	Somewhat strong
5	Strong
6	
7	Very strong
8	
9	
10	Very, very strong (almost maximum)

	Monday	Tuesday	Wednesday	Thursday	Friday	Saturday	Sunday
6.30							
7.00							
7.30							
8.00							
8.30							
9.00							
9.30							
10.00							
10.30							
11.00							
11.30							
12.00							
12.30							
1.00							
1.30							
2.00							
2.30							
3.00							
3.30							
4.00							
4.30							
5.00							
5.30							
6.00							
6.30							
7.00							
7.30							
8.00							
8.30							
9.00							
9.30							
10.00							
10.30							
11.00							

Appendix 13: Documentation of follow up sessions

Name:	Date:
Date of appointment:	
Diagnosis:	
Key Symptoms:	
New Medical Information:	
Progress (circle): *Resolved / Improved / Minor improvement / No change / Deteriorated*	
Previous Therapy:	
Outcome Measures: e.g. Leicester Cough Questionnaire Score, or Maximum Phonation Time	
Vocal Hygiene:	
Practicing (circle):	*Yes / No / Sometimes*
Practicing exercises correctly (circle):	*Yes / Partially / No*
If no – specify:	
Implementing exercises at first sign of cough (circle): *Yes / No / Sometimes*	
Exercises given today:	
Advice given today:	
Impression:	

Index

CPSIA information can be obtained
at www.ICGtesting.com
Printed in the USA
BVOW10s2109200516

448964BV00001B/1/P